Praise for *The Open Heart Companion*

"*The Open Heart Companion* is just that—a book that acts as a loving, wise, and comforting partner who gently guides you through the stages of preparing for and successfully completing open-heart surgery. A life-saving gift filled with invaluable resources, real-life stories, and must-know information, this book is required reading for all patients and loved ones."

—**Cheryl Richardson**
Author of *Take Time for Your Life: A Personal Coach's 7-Step Program for Creating the Life You Want*

"*The Open Heart Companion* is *must* reading for anyone who requires open-heart surgery. Written by a life coach who has been there herself, it will help you get the most out of this dramatic and life-changing experience."

—**Christiane Northrup, MD**
Author of *Women's Bodies, Women's Wisdom: Creating Physical and Emotional Health and Healing*

"This passionate and personal guide will help you both survive and thrive after open-heart surgery."

—**Mehmet C. Oz, MD**
Pioneering heart surgeon and author of *Healing from the Heart: A Leading Surgeon Combines Eastern and Western Traditions to Create the Medicine of the Future*

"This beautifully written, comprehensive, and absolutely accurate account of how to go into, come out of, and recover from open-heart surgery is a must for patients and physicians alike. I plan to keep a supply on hand for my own patients, confident that they will find it, as I did, immensely instructive and helpful."

—**Marianne J. Legato, MD**
Author of *The Female Heart: The Truth about Women and Heart Disease*

"Maggie Lichtenberg has created a terrific resource for those undergoing open-heart surgery, both for the preparation and the recovery period. Drawn from dozens of patient and caregiver interviews, the book is filled with specific exercises and insights to make the open-heart experience easier on the patient and loved ones."

—**Amy Verstappen**
President, Adult Congenital Heart Association

THE OPEN HEART COMPANION

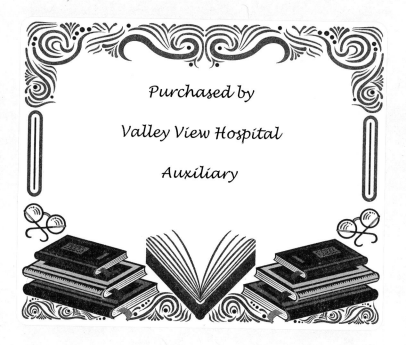

Purchased by

Valley View Hospital

Auxiliary

The
OPEN HEART
Companion

Preparation and Guidance

for Open-Heart Surgery Recovery

MAGGIE LICHTENBERG, PCC

Foreword by Kathleen Blake, MD

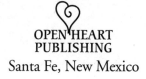

OPEN HEART
PUBLISHING

Santa Fe, New Mexico

Open Heart Publishing
4 Cosmos Court, Santa Fe, NM 87508
www.openheartcoach.com

Book and cover design by Janice St. Marie
Cover photograph by Bart Sadowski

Printed in Canada

*Disclaimer: The content in this book is not intended as a substitute for medical
or professional advice. Readers are encouraged to consult their physician on all
health matters, especially symptoms that may require professional diagnosis or
medical attention.*

Library of Congress Cataloging-in-Publication Data

Lichtenberg, Maggie K.

The open heart companion : preparation and guidance for open-heart
surgery recovery / Maggie Lichtenberg. -- 1st ed. -- Santa Fe,
N.M. : Open Heart Publishing, 2006.

p. ; cm.
ISBN-13: 978-0-97760-630-6
ISBN-10: 0-9776063-0-9
Includes glossary and resource directory.
Includes bibliographical references and index.

1. Heart--Surgery--Patients--Rehabilitation. 2. Heart--Surgery--
Patients--Counseling. 3. Heart--Surgery--Psychological aspects.
4. Postoperative care. 5. Rehabilitation counseling. I. Title.

RD598 .L53 2006   2005937557
617.4/12--dc22   0606

10 9 8 7 6 5 4 3 2 1

For Bill, my partner in life,
whose love and encouragement
are always there

Contents

PART ONE
What to Do Before Your Date with Open-Heart Surgery

Foreword

NO ONE *WANTS* TO HAVE HEART SURGERY, but over 700,000 potentially life-saving open-heart operations are performed every year in the United States. For each of the courageous and apprehensive individuals who undergo cardiac surgery there is a surrounding network of spouses, partners, children, friends, and colleagues, which means that open-heart procedures directly and indirectly change the lives of several million people in this country every year.

Symptoms of heart disease can develop gradually or suddenly, and so the time available to prepare for heart surgery varies enormously from person to person. For some patients—and their families—this will require a decision to be made within days, or even minutes, in the context of an unforeseen medical emergency, and it may be their first experience with surgery of any kind. For others, since heart disease can run in a family, confronting the prospect may awaken memories of an operation performed on a loved one years ago, when the field was new, options were limited, and risks were generally higher than they are today. Every cardiac patient comes to this experience with their own unique life history behind them and with their own strengths and challenges, hopes and fears.

A cardiac patient's team includes physicians, nurses, and other essential, highly experienced staff. These are individuals who have chosen to commit themselves to fixing broken hearts because they are driven to make a difference in the lives of patients entrusted to their care. Not uncommonly they too have had a personal or family experience with serious illness, one that strengthens their resolve to help others in similar distress. But the medical members of the patient's team have also acquired a familiarity and comfort with cardiac procedures that is not shared by the layperson. In fact, it is their very experience and ease with these procedures that make it possible for medical professionals to do this work calmly and competently; in almost all circumstances we proceed with a high level of confidence that the vast majority of our patients will do well in the long run. Simultaneously, however, we must remember that for our patients this is a journey into new, unfamiliar, and frightening territory.

For all of these reasons, the need for a guidebook is obvious and compelling—and this is what Maggie Lichtenberg has provided, through her research and by generously sharing her own experience with us. This is a personal and passionate book in which the author describes a history of living with heart disease, her eventual decision to undergo open-heart surgery to correct a rare congenital valve condition, and her recovery from the operation. Based on her skills as a coach and writer, she has designed a plan that can be used by those who anticipate or have recently undergone *any* major medical or surgical event. Informed preoperative decision-making is strongly and wisely recommended. A compelling case is made for active enlistment of medical professionals, family, and friends in the recovery process, and many different options for relaxation and recuperation are presented. Most importantly, the challenge of dealing with unexpected ups and downs after surgery is honestly discussed.

No amount of preparation before surgery can address every eventual question or concern. Questions often rise to the surface in response to one's personal experience. Rather than attempt to answer all questions and address all possible situations, Maggie Lichtenberg focuses on how to get help and information when needed.

Though she is careful to remind the reader that she is not a healthcare professional, her book should be a guide for all medical professionals who hope to understand their patients and meet their needs. Because it outlines a series of plans for thoughtful and collaborative action, it will be equally useful for those assisting in the care of a family member or friend. And finally, I am grateful to at last have a guide I can recommend not just to my patients and their families but also to my medical and nursing colleagues as we strive to improve the care our patients receive.

KATHLEEN BLAKE, MD
CARDIOLOGIST
PRESIDENT, NEW MEXICO HEART INSTITUTE

How to Use This Book

SINCE MY PERSONAL ENCOUNTER with open-heart surgery two and a half years ago, I have felt a powerful calling to write about my experience in order to support others in preparing for such an ordeal and, in particular, in making better plans for the recovery period than I did. The simple truth is that whether you have had—or will have—coronary artery bypass surgery, a valve replacement or repair, or even a heart transplant, as with any procedure requiring the opening of the sternum you will have weeks, maybe months, in front of you before recouping your full strength and well-being. My commitment to patients and caregivers alike is to prepare you for the practical realities and repercussions of any open-heart surgery, emergency or elective.

I care deeply about this subject because although I was well prepared to undergo the surgical event itself, I paid little attention to the fact that there even *was* a recovery period. After all, I was basically strong and healthy! But while I was careful to find experts to help me prepare for surgery, there was no guardian angel of guidance at the other end to educate and reassure me through the seemingly endless weeks of fatigue, episodes of depression, and other setbacks that unnecessarily prolonged my healing. I had to remind myself, over and over, "The operative word here is 'temporary.' You *will* fully recover."

Along the way, I compiled a "wish-I-knew-beforehand" list that I used as the basis for developing—with the help of medical professionals and fellow cardiac surgery patients—the information and specific planning guidelines I share with you here. Knowing what I now know, I see there are serious stumbling blocks that can be avoided. Advance knowledge, simply, is power.

Part I of this book covers preparation for surgery, Part II discusses what happens in the hospital, and Part III addresses recovery. The **Guidelines and Checklists** section at the end of the book is intended to help you structure your planning throughout. If you wish, save my personal story, set forth in the Prologue, for a later time and go directly to the part of the book that's most relevant right now—Part I, for instance, if your surgery is imminent, or Part III if you are newly home from the hospital. Feel free to bounce around pursuing topics that seem most relevant to you, because my aim is to help you plan your own course of action. Toward that end I have provided a detailed table of contents. But I also hope you will explore the entire book thoroughly, because every bit of information included in it connects with the whole.

Two caveats: I am not a trained health professional. I am a thriving layperson who experienced open-heart surgery. And so with every pivotal medical issue discussed I will be steering you to the appropriate medical professional. Second, I have not been able to highlight every potential concern. Nevertheless, I believe the information presented here—drawing on my own experience and that of dozens of open-heart patients and their caregivers whom I've talked with, and on my research and conversations with medical professionals—covers the most important issues. I have provided both a **Glossary** and a **Resources** section at the back of the book to help you find further sources of advice and support.

Finally, my intention is to help you envelop yourself in a positive, proactive frame of mind during the rugged bad days and nights ahead, as well as during the times that bring a breath of fresh air, for they too will be there! Whether you have time now, before your procedure, to design a recovery plan, or are already convalescing, it is my fervent hope that the advice that follows will educate and support you through a good outcome and a speedier, less stressful recovery.

My Own Journey
from Resistance to Action

Soul loves the journey in itself.

—DAVID WHYTE

OPEN-HEART SURGERY PRESENTS unique challenges. The heart—which some would say is the cradle for the soul as well as a muscular organ—is exposed and disturbed. During an open-heart operation the breastbone is divided, then the protective sack around the heart is cut open. The heart lies naked, most often stilled as its functions are turned over to a heart-lung machine for several hours while arteries are reconfigured or valves repaired or replaced. Does the essence of the heart's experience during surgery permanently change us? We may never know. Yet we surely can acknowledge that the very existence of open-heart surgery, in all its variants, is a miracle.

My Heart Story

I was diagnosed at birth with a mild version of Ebstein's Anomaly, a condition so minor it was never supposed to interfere with my life. I believed for years that my congenital heart defect, a slight structural valve displacement, would never become symptomatic, never stop me from doing all that lay ahead in my future. And indeed, I went on to live a personally and professionally productive life in high gear well into my adult years.

During that time I wasn't what one would call spiritually conscious. I didn't examine much in depth. I didn't ask the big questions. I had no religious leanings. I was busy, busy, busy—raising a family, overcoming a divorce, and forging a career in New York publishing.

Then at age fifty-three, seven years after moving from New York City to Boston, Massachusetts, I had my first encounter with arrhythmia, irregular heartbeat. The problem, called atrial flutter, wasn't serious, I was assured, and it responded quickly to a standard medication. All in all, I still viewed myself as a very healthy person.

Fortunately, learning to meditate two years earlier, in 1993, had profoundly changed my life. Searching for an antidote to my increasingly stressful professional life, I had begun to frequent a health spa to get back in touch with myself, to reconnect with my natural joy for living. I chose Canyon Ranch in Lenox, in the Berkshires, because I had wonderfully happy memories of childhood summer camp in that part of the country. There I could plan programs to thoroughly enjoy myself, to hike in the mountains, eat exceptional nutritious meals, have a daily massage, and try out new activities, like tai chi and meditation. Not only did I relish the peace and calm I captured by meditating upon waking up in the morning then again before my evening meal, but the cumulative effect of practicing this discipline twice a day seemed to open up my life. From this expansion I learned to focus inside as well as on the outside.

Does escaping to a health spa sound simply trendy and indulgent? At the time, my ample paycheck had been going straight to the bank as a direct deposit. I was so busy at work—so identified with my job as marketing director for a book publishing company—that the idea of "getting a life" beyond that hadn't caught up with me. And, as it turned out, my expensive five-day sojourns at the spa did in fact set the stage for authentic self-discovery. The day I first decided to try a health spa, I remember so clearly, I had come home from work, looked in the mirror, and asked the face that looked back at me, "Is this *it?* There *must* be more than this." There must be more possibility for fulfillment out there, I thought, more purpose to my life than merely accumulating a pile of money that sits in a bank.

That questioning moment was the beginning of my heart journey.

However odd it may sound, it wasn't until the death of a beloved elderly cat in 1994 that I reached a new level of spiritual awareness, the discovery deep inside that my being was profoundly connected to, and part of, an infinite intelligence—call that God or Spirit or the Divine.

It happened like this. I adored my little kitty and refused to acknowledge that she was dying. Instead, I hired a young veterinary technician to come to the house daily to administer fluids via injection beneath her tight skin. Lionhearted was eighteen and ready to let go. Yet it was difficult for me to help her do that until I was told of a compassionate vet who would come to the house to perform euthanasia. Finally I called him and made a date for two days later. By now Lionhearted was spending her days sitting stone-still facing the back of a living-room chair, avoiding my gaze altogether, even when I sat down for my evening meditation on the couch beside her.

The vet came. As I gently stroked my beloved feline companion, he put her to sleep. I wept buckets. I also knew I had made the best decision.

The next day the revelation occurred. I used to walk to work in Boston, a brisk, twenty-five-minute stroll that included smiling my way past eight bronze duckling sculptures, a tribute to award-winning children's book author Robert McCloskey, in the Boston Public Garden, traversing the four-lane concrete expanse of Charles Street, and then proceeding through Boston Common up to my office on Beacon Hill. That day, still tearful, I looked up and saw that the treetops were glistening. Drawn in more and more by the sparkle of the sun on the waving branches, all the treetops seemingly merged into an entire chorus of undulating leaves shimmering with peace and delight, I stood still in my tracks. I was unable to avert my gaze and move on up the hill. Lionhearted was everywhere! Her spirit had rejoined nature's awesome whole in a dancing medley of light. She was beaming out love all over me.

In the fall of 1994, curious to pursue my insight on the Common, I said to myself, "Let's try the original place, Canyon Ranch in Tucson." There, enveloped in the beauty and the late afternoon fall light of Arizona, I experienced another moving revelation during a walking meditation. As I watched the purple majesty of a sunset over the Tucson mountains, in that instant I felt the Southwest calling to me. I stood in awe, transfixed. I could live here! I could immerse myself in this beauty daily! I did not understand where the message was coming from, or why I should receive such a calling. Then, that evening, I meandered into one of the after-dinner talks given by a person who identified himself as a coach. "Who is this 'coach,'" I wondered, "who has nothing to do with sports?" But a mere two hours later I had been thoroughly introduced to the emerging career of personal and professional life coaching, and I had hired this man to support me in designing a new life for myself.

I returned home to Boston for the time being, but the messages from the Southwest were too potent to ignore. Within six months I had changed every aspect of my existence. I ended a long-term intimate relationship. I resigned from my job, enrolled in an international coach training program, and laid plans to reconfigure my career. I addressed the nagging but minor issue of my atrial flutter by having a cardioversion—a simple, nonsurgical, morning-in-the-hospital procedure—which seemed to correct the problem altogether. Then I left dear family and lifelong friends, and two twenty-something grown children, and, without a partner, moved two thousand miles across the country. Although Canyon Ranch is in Tucson, I didn't consider moving to Arizona because for six months of the year Arizona is simply too hot. Instead I was drawn to four-season Santa Fe, where I was to experience daily the invigorating natural beauty of Northern New Mexico and satisfy my dormant longing for living closer to nature.

Seven deeply fulfilling years in Santa Fe followed. I established my own practice as a coach, eventually drawing on my experience in publishing to specialize in working with people in that field. I met the man whom I recognized as my soul partner in life. We married in July 2000 and together built a contemporary pueblo-style home.

Warnings and Reprieves

My first two years in Santa Fe were incident free as far as even minor cardiac symptoms were concerned, in spite of the 7,000-foot altitude. With Bill, my new-found soul mate but not yet my husband, I hiked the many byways of the Windsor Trail, whose trailhead marker stands at a lofty 10,400 feet above sea level. We would climb from there up to the saddle, stopping to take in the light shimmering through silvery-green aspen treetops. The intense blue sky spilled outward, way, way beyond—an infinity pathway. We'd pause and silently beam ourselves up through the tree-tops, feeling deeply a part of the oneness.

Often we would continue up to Raven's Ridge, reaching an altitude of more than 11,000 feet, and there we'd eat our packed lunch: two meat-and-salad sandwiches, an extra peanut-butter-and-jelly sandwich for Bill, sometimes a hard-boiled egg or two, grapes, cookies, trail mix, and lots and lots of water. Brave gray-and-white piñon jays eagerly helped with the crumbs, sometimes right out of my hand. Raven's Ridge looks across a lush green valley to Baldy, Santa Fe's highest peak at 12,466 feet. It is a spectacular location. As a rumpled sign posted on a piñon tree suggests, I too dream that my ashes may be scattered to the gentle winds from Raven's Ridge one day, when my "time of transition" comes.

Then, in the fall of 1997, the atrial flutter returned. I was annoyed since it had been "corrected" two years before, in Boston. My first Santa Fe cardiologist—whose specialty happened to be pediatric Ebstein's—gently warned that one day I might need to have the valve in question repaired. In his words, the "status of the tricuspid valve" was making the right atrium "irritable," or, to put it another way, highly susceptible to arrhythmias. I knew that repair would mean a huge surgery, and I quickly dismissed the possibility.

In the meantime, radio frequency ablation had been invented, a procedure designed to ablate (i.e., delete) the flutter's pathway in the heart so that the heart's electrical system would be forced back into the normal sinus rhythm circuit. My new cardiologist referred me to an EP, an electrophysiologist, at the New Mexico Heart Institute in Albuquerque, to perform the ablation and so fix me "forever." After two ablations three months apart, that particular arrhythmia was indeed permanently put to rest.

Again I was home free! Again I took up the physical activities that gave me so much pleasure: more hiking, more cross-country skiing. I was not on medication of any kind. I had no worries. I was able to lead a blessed life as before.

In late November 1999, at age fifty-seven, however, I experienced the first episode of what felt like an entirely new kind of disturbance. Initially I ignored it, even when it happened again. But eventually it recurred often enough that in the spring of 2002 I asked my cardiologist for a heart monitor, which captured an episode of atrial fibrillation on tape just as it was happening. "Atrial fib"—what was *that* all about?

For me it meant severe, painful throat constriction (rather than the more common racing heartbeat) that would immobilize me for a couple of hours before my heart reverted back to a normal rhythm. These episodes occurred very sporadically; that first year I had only three. Then they began to happen every three months, then every three weeks. The primary manifestation around the throat would be so painful that I could not lie down in a prone position. The pattern became increasingly nocturnal, so any night this happened I was forced to remain upright. This meant no sleeping. So

I would read. I tried meditating. I tried Korean yogic deep-breathing exercises. I was given several new medications that didn't agree with me, nor did they work.

What began to get my attention was the increasing frequency and severity of these attacks. In October 2002, my coaching colleague, Sandra, and I were on a business trip attending the Seventh Annual Conference of the International Coach Federation in Atlanta, Georgia. The night before our presentation titled "How to Marry Publishing and Speaking Success," I woke up at 3 a.m. with that all-too-familiar constriction of the throat. I had been awakened by an episode of fib three weeks earlier, but the one before that had been three *months* before. This made me crazy. Here I was once again driven upright, forced to wait it out. But this time I was in a convention hotel's double bed, propped against pillows in the middle of the night, dreading the truth. I imagined having to check myself into an Atlanta hospital. I thought of asking Bill's brother and sister-in-law, who lived nearby, which hospital to go to. Finally, I faced the prospect of not being able to deliver my presentation unless the debilitating arrhythmia went away. It did revert back to normal as the day dawned, and by 2 p.m. I had stabilized and was able to deliver the presentation with Sandra—but just barely.

This was the moment of truth that spirited me back to San Antonio, Texas, to my original EP, who had performed the ablations five years earlier. Somewhere deep inside me I knew these increasingly frequent occurrences of atrial fib were not casual, unrelated medical annoyances. The attacks were getting my attention, raising my awareness to acknowledge an as yet unclear but profound development occurring inside my physical vessel. The irregular rhythms beating in my heart were trying to tell me, You need help! A mystery is stirring inside your heart, I acknowledged to myself. *Love* your heart. Find out what's going on.

In San Antonio, Dr. Machell temporarily soothed my fears. No, I would not want to put myself through the major surgery of repairing the tricuspid valve. He was also iffy about going the pacemaker route. He wanted me to focus on drug therapy as *the* panacea. He put me back on the anti-arrhythmic Propafenone (also known as Rythmol), which I had tolerated well before, in Boston. Any time an episode of fib came on, he advised me, I should take a double dose, followed by a second, lower dose an hour later. If that didn't bleep it out, he recommended going back to my standard three-times-a-day 150 mg dosage. During that consultation Dr. Machell did not, however, order an echocardiogram—a simple sound-wave test imaging the heart. I had not had an echo in five years. Looking back, I wish I had understood at the time the importance of taking the initiative to *request* one; if I had done so, the progression of my increasingly "leaky" tricuspid valve would have been immediately and blatantly apparent. But—as we find out in stages while navigating our way through complicated medical challenges—most medical specialists will think first of approaching the problem from within their own areas of expertise.

In the meantime, for a while after returning to Santa Fe I didn't need the anti-arrhythmic medicine. Three months passed. Nothing! I had this thing licked, I told myself.

The Handwriting on the Wall

In February 2003 the fib came back. At first Dr. Machell's on-the-spot dosage scheme worked beautifully. The onset of fibrillation usually began around midnight. I just had to be very patient for two hours until my heart rhythm would revert. I began with 225 mg of Propafenone, then swallowed another 150 mg an hour later. Yes, I sat upright in pain, trying to read, trying to pass that first hour. Then usually somewhere within the second hour I could lie down again. This was the beginning of a period of losing several nights of sleep, for weeks. Fortunately Bill could slumber through all of this. He always encouraged me to wake him if I needed to, but I chose not to. Sleep deprivation was not a quality of life I wanted to inflict on anyone else, let alone my husband.

In March 2003 I flew to Wilmington, North Carolina, to present a workshop at the Southeast Coaching Conference. My presentation and role at the conference went well, and two hours after it ended I had a little time to pass before going to the airport. I set out to walk along the city's beautiful riverbank. Out of nowhere that I could fathom, a powerful attack suddenly stopped me dead in my tracks. For a few minutes it felt like the old fib, then it segued into a feeling of exhaustion. My reaction once again was outrage. How could this keep happening to me, especially when I was away from home? Was I particularly stressed? I didn't think so. I struggled to come up with an answer, a reason, and of course I couldn't.

At a snail's pace I walked back to the hotel, stopping every five or ten steps. Where the sidewalk inclined slightly, I had to struggle harder. I made it back to the hotel and boarded the shuttle van with my coaching colleague, Rachelle. We sought out a café at the airport before proceeding to our departure gate. I did not tell Rachelle what was going on.

From Wilmington, I was on my way to New York City to make a quick stop to see my two-year-old grandson, my son and daughter-in-law, and my daughter and her partner. But once on the plane bound for La Guardia, I knew I couldn't navigate the airport and the cab ride to Washington Heights—indeed, it might have been dangerous to try. Before the plane took off I pulled out my cell phone, called my daughter, and asked her to meet me at the airport. I was frightened, and rightly so. Once safely in Manhattan, it took twenty-four hours for the abnormal conduction pathway to right itself, miserably straining my visit.

I was still thinking of my fib episodes as a management problem, that they could be dealt with by calling on my new regimen of on-the-spot heavy doses of Propafenone—I was in charge! But maybe, a little voice whispered, I needed to establish a relationship with a new EP closer to home than Texas, just in case. I was given a referral to a highly recommended doctor by a close friend of Bill's, but I would have to wait a month to get in to see her.

In the meantime, I was determined to carry on as usual. In April, I went back to New York, this time with Bill for a preplanned home exchange visit. One evening my entire side of the family and I, nine of us, were dining together at a Chinese restaurant in the West Village when *whap!*—the fib hit again, smack in between the dumplings and the moo shoo pork with pancakes. For some reason I couldn't put my finger on, it was comforting that all the people who are most important to me were with me that night. I only understood why when we were reunited three months later in decidedly different circumstances.

Finally, in early May 2003, I had my first appointment with Dr. Kathleen Blake at the New Mexico Heart Institute in Albuquerque. She wanted to start our new relationship by locking in the atrial fibrillation diagnosis on paper, and again I was given a heart monitor. The next time an episode of atrial fib came on, I was to attach two small electrodes to my chest, record the rhythm on the heart monitor (which is the size of a Walkman), then call an 800 number and transmit the recording over the phone. Since I was now having atrial fib every two or three nights, I did not have to wait long to confirm my symptoms on tape. Dr. Blake also ordered an echocardiogram, and once those results came in, she made a case for the severity of the progression of my Ebstein's. I was experiencing a conduction problem, she told me; once again, my heart's electrical signals were traveling along an abnormal pathway. One repair route, she suggested, could include the insertion of a new kind of pacemaker to regulate my heart rhythms. But before she would proceed with a pacemaker, she insisted I first seek out a consultation with the Ebstein's experts at the Mayo Clinic in Rochester, Minnesota.

This was serious stuff. My predicament *did* have to do with being an Ebsteiner, and at age sixty-one I could no longer avoid the fact that my condition was becoming progressively worse. No matter that for decades I had believed my Ebstein's was so mild I would never be physically limited, let alone need surgical repair. The writing was on the wall, the ink long dry.

Overcoming Resistance and Choosing My Best Option
I had a five-week wait in front of me before I could consult with the doctors at the Mayo Clinic. In the meantime, I continued to curb the episodes of fib with heavy medication, but once again they were happening more frequently, and I would sometimes be depleted for entire days afterward. I had a decision to make. I was scheduled for another business trip, to Los Angeles, to participate in the annual Publishers Marketing Association's University, for which I was to moderate two panels, and to attend the annual book convention Book Expo America. Should I make this business trip or gracefully let it go?

In the end, I didn't want to give it up. It was just too important to me professionally. I knew my nights could be rough, but my daytimes were usually clear. I decided to enlist a support structure and go for it. I invited a colleague who was planning to attend anyway, to share my hotel room at the Wilshire Grand for the first couple of nights. I asked my husband to pop over to L.A. for the rest. That way I would have caring people near me if I ran into trouble. I also arranged for two of my fellow panelists to become instant substitute moderators in the event I'd be unable to lead the panels myself. If eighty percent of my five days in Los Angeles were good ones, I figured, I would consider the trip worthwhile.

I was lucky. During my first two days in L.A. I felt fine. My third day was terrible; I had to give up my participation on the second panel. But the fourth day, the opening of the BEA, was excellent; I had many fortuitous meetings with publishing folk both known and unknown, and energetic excursions around the massive Los Angeles convention floor. The last day I also scored as a good one, but I was definitely wearying by the time Bill and I flew home.

Back in Santa Fe, a little less than a week before my scheduled consultations at the Mayo Clinic, I was visited by a brainstorm. Why was I waiting for the siege—for the onset of fib during the night—before taking the large dose of anti-arrhythmic medicine? Why not take it *before* I went to bed? So I followed my instinct and began taking the medication an hour before bedtime every evening, and for the next five nights I had no recurrences. Again I seemed to have conquered the fib!

The electrophysiologist at the Mayo seemed impressed by my story. "That's a very encouraging sign for you," he observed. "You are in fact a miracle sitting in front of me. You have already lived thirty years longer than any adult with Ebstein's I know of before becoming symptomatic. Maybe surgery isn't in the cards for you at this time, but let's just see what the adult congenital cardiologist and the Ebstein's surgeon have to say."

Had the EP reviewed my echocardiogram? I wondered. Was this another reprieve, or was he just softening the blow? I don't know to this day, but when I met with the adult congenital cardiologist and the surgeon they each confirmed what Dr. Blake had reported to my deaf ears a month earlier. The "regurgitation" or backlash of blood circulating back through the tricuspid valve had now progressed to "severe" levels. My infamous tricuspid valve now presented as severe Ebstein's, a valve so leaky that it needed to be repaired or replaced. That this scenario for major surgery seemed to occur overnight continued to infuriate me.

But it wasn't sudden, of course. I had become symptomatic eight years before, I had just refused to connect the arrhythmias to that long-ago childhood diagnosis. I had chosen to believe instead that my new symptoms represented a different—and minor—problem. I had traveled to the Mayo Clinic hoping to get away with a pacemaker at the very most, but it was impressed upon me again and again that there was no point in putting in a pacemaker until the tricuspid valve could be made to close properly. Their recommendation: I should take care of this in the next month or two. That meant open-heart surgery.

I'm exceptionally lucky that I had time to prepare myself for the operation. It's a double whammy when you have to go in on an emergency basis. I picked a date five weeks out—July 16, 2003—a date deliberately beyond the two-week Cape Cod family vacation Bill and I had planned. All my kids were there: my son and daughter-in-law, my daughter and her partner, and our two-year-old grandson, Zev. (It was that summer that Zev met, and became impassioned by, The Beach.)

I felt very strong and very happy during those two weeks. My regimen of preempting atrial fib with a dose of anti-arrhythmic every night worked a hundred percent. Did I really need this operation? I wondered. I felt so well on the Cape that I considered my healing had already begun, and I made this point often, to myself and others, while also acknowledging that, yes, I was experiencing shortness of breath from time to time. In fact, at this point the slightest incline under foot made me uncomfortable.

One key resource for me was the discovery of Peggy Huddleston's program, set forth in her book *Prepare for Surgery, Heal Faster* and its accompanying tape. While on the Cape, I played the twenty-minute tape twice a day and found it invaluable. It's primarily a relaxation tape, with guided visualizations to focus on desired outcomes after surgery, and it helped me enormously to move beyond my fears about the surgery and *believe* in a positive outcome. I had become confident and calm. I was ready.

During those vacation weeks my daughter-in-law, Meredith, asked me if I had arranged for caregivers and domestic help. I hadn't. The depth of my denial reared its head again. I'd be fine, and after all, I had Bill as my staunch ally. On everyone's urging, for Bill's sake as well as mine, I emailed one of my closest friends back in Santa Fe to ask if she would organize what I've come to call a "home team." Some friends could come by to help with household chores, bring dinner, run an errand, or just to visit for a few minutes. I remember how hard it was for me to ask for this, yet I did. (I also woefully underestimated my recovery time. Two weeks of dinner delivery was by no means enough coverage. Little did I know that in my case it would be six to eight weeks before I'd make significant strides toward recovery.)

My Date with Open-Heart Surgery

The patient education department of the Mayo Clinic, like those of many hospitals, provides an excellent presurgery videotape, *Your Heart Surgery: What to Expect, What You Can Do.* Before leaving for Minnesota for my surgery, Bill and I watched the fifteen-minute video at home. It chronicles the progress of events from a patient's arrival at the hospital the day before the operation through the first week afterward. It includes footage shot inside the ICU and shows the patient hooked up to a heart-lung machine. I found the image of that machine astonishing. It seemed huge. That thing is going to be my lifeline! I thought to myself. The script tries to be as reassuring as possible, of course, as we follow the patient through his next several days: sitting up now, less tubing evident, not thrilled with the first hospital meal with which he is presented. He's up and walking very soon, support hose visible, smiling at his visitors and dutifully coughing several times a day into a small plastic device.

The video could not have been gentler. Yet it left me anxious. I knew it was good for me to have at least a big-picture summary of what was to come. Still, a part of me could not believe I was about to go through with this.

I was particularly obsessed with whether or not I would need a blood transfusion and, if so, whether I should provide my own blood in advance. To get answers to these and other nitty-gritty questions I'd been too numb to ask when I had my initial consultation with my surgeon, I prepared and faxed fourteen questions to his secretary and made a phone date to speak with him.

Yes, my surgeon told me, there is a seventy-five percent chance that an Ebstein's patient will need a blood transfusion. (Many open-heart patients do not, my physician's assistant at the Mayo told me later, because in many kinds of surgeries the patient's own blood is retrieved, filtered, and returned as much as possible.) And, the surgeon continued, if a transfusion becomes necessary, more blood is needed than can be furnished by the individual. Additionally, if you are prone to atrial fibrillation most likely you will have been on an anticoagulant like Coumadin. That adds a complexity. All things considered, my surgeon advised me to give my own blood in advance only if I felt strongly about doing so. In the end, because additional blood would have to be mixed with my own anyway, I chose not to. As it turned out, I did not need a blood transfusion.

Do you need to break bones in order to get in to operate on the heart? I asked. If so, which ones, how many, and how long is the healing process for the bones specifically?

"First of all," my surgeon answered, "we don't use the words *break* or *chop*." Then he assured me that he was one of the surgeons who performs "limited access incisions." In my case, the breastbone (sternum) would be divided down the center through an incision made two inches below its top, then wired back up after the operation was completed. He knew, he said, that women in particular tend to be sensitive about a scar showing if they wear V-neck garments, and he would aim to keep the incision as low as possible. The bone would heal completely in six to eight weeks, and scarring would be minimal. That all sounded horrifying, but what could I do? Slowly I segued into acceptance.

I was also concerned about being on, then coming off, a ventilator (breathing device) after the operation. I had read that coming out of anesthesia, having the tube removed, and being prompted to breathe on one's own again is a significant challenge for the patient. That, combined with the thought of being trapped on my back, restricted from turning from side to side, worried me. I am prone to a chronic midback spasm condition, avoidable only if I am able to stay off my back, I explained. What could I be given for pain during that time?

My surgeon's answer was not very satisfying. I would be on a general painkiller anyway, and if one medication didn't work, the anesthesia people in the ICU would be "experimenting with alternatives." "Unfortunately," he added, "so many of the painkillers have a nauseating effect." Failing everything, they would consult the Mayo Clinic's pain service.

We continued through my list of questions (and a few others that just popped into my head), covering my fear of allergic reactions, revisiting the pros and cons of replacement valves and success rates after right-sided Maze procedures (an additional rhythm-correcting procedure I had agreed to), and ending with more mundane concerns, like when would I be able to raise my arms to wash my own hair. The answers were sometimes disturbing, but I took it all in. And, at a certain point, I realized I just needed to let go and trust that the decision I was making would lead to positive results in the long run.

As my date with open-heart surgery approached, Bill and I flew to Minnesota from New Mexico and installed ourselves in one of the reasonably priced hotel suites across the street from the hospital. My son would be coming from New York to stay there with Bill during my week in the hospital. And my daughter and her partner would be arriving a day later.

The next day, the prerequisite coronary angiogram was performed. A catheter was inserted through my wrist vein into the heart, to make sure nothing else was going on (like a blockage) besides my structural valve displacement and accompanying "severe regurgitation." My angiogram was normal: green light to proceed. That afternoon I met again with my surgeon. He was most reassuring (of course), even breezy.

Then the day of the surgery itself arrived. I checked in at the appointed location at 5:30 a.m. We were asked if we would like a visit from a chaplain, after which a gentle uniformed elder held our hands while reciting a nondenominational prayer. We were touched and soothed. Then the gurney and the gurney navigator arrived, swooshing me off, sitting upright and cross-legged, on a long meandering route to the pre-op waiting area.

There some twenty patients on gurneys were lying prone, flat and silent. We were all lined up in a row, as in the children's book about Madeleine, barely inches from each other. I felt out of place sitting up and gazing down at all the subdued bodies, but I was also a little proud of myself for being so conscious and positive. I had declined the sedative for this waiting period because I wanted to be fully alert in order to review headset instructions and the affirmations I wanted someone on the OR team to read to me as I went under.

I was lucky to have a short wait; ten minutes later they were ready for me. Still upright and cross-legged, I was wheeled into an extremely well-lit and bustling operating room. The adrenalin flow was palpable. Without pause, the team of attendants moved me from the gurney to a skinny sliver of a table and began to strap me down. "Wait!" I protested. "I need to go over my affirmation requests and my music with one of you first! And I need to delay lying flat on my back as long as I can because I have a chronic back issue."

The team, ready to get moving, looked surprised at how alert and intentional I was, but together we worked out who would read the affirmations and who would take my Walkman earphones on and off during the operation. Then I had to lie down. IVs were inserted in both arms at once. My back began to hurt. "Here goes," someone said. And that was that.

I spent four hours in surgery, my heart functions parked on the heart-lung machine while my tricuspid valve was repaired. I don't remember much about my approximately twenty-four hours in the ICU, and perhaps that's a good thing. (I had heard about ICU amnesia from other heart patients beforehand.) For the most part, I must have been happily blanked out. What I do remember is an experience of high stress coming off the ventilator. Not only did my cerebral brain seem disoriented, but my reptilian counterpart was resisting letting go of the device, although letting go is necessary to complete the return to normal breathing. Those dangling few minutes were tough, but I also remember a soothing, reassuring nurse's voice softly speaking in my ear: "It's okay, Maggie. It's okay, Maggie. Just breathe normally. Breathe normally..."

When I woke up the next day in my hospital room, my loved ones were around me, beaming. I was ecstatic. I had made it through! I was there! Alive! And kicking! I felt tremendous relief and release. The unit nurse was cheery too as she gave me my first lesson in turning around in bed, and getting in and out. No arms—use elbows only! "Have a little visit with everyone," she said. "Then I recommend a delicious two-hour nap. Your visitors can come back when you get your lunch, and after that you'll have another two-hour nap. Then we'll get you up for a little walk. You're going to have a wonderful day!"

All things considered, I had a very positive hospital experience. A different day-nurse was assigned to me for each of my seven days, and all of them were terrific: focused, caring, cheerful, highly skilled, and easy to talk to. In the "expect good days and bad days" department, I passed one miserable night barely able to get my nurse's attention because she was so occupied with a patient next door. Night nurses, I discovered, were far more pressured because more patients seemed to develop serious issues at night. (My erstwhile neighbor, in fact, had taken such a turn for the worse that night that the nurse returned her to the ICU.)

I knew to give up expecting to sleep well from the start. With chest drainage tubes still attached to my abdomen, a heavy twenty-four-hour heart monitor strapped to me, and various measurements—blood tests, blood pressure, temperature, and more—necessary around the clock, turning into a cat-napper was the only way to go. Giddy with happiness to be on the other side of my operation, I saw details of discomfort as just that—details.

My husband and my children were an incredible comfort to me during that week. They walked up and down the halls with me. They encouraged me to eat. They were attentive to exactly what was going on, proactive advocates for my support. Most of all, I had made it through my surgery with flying colors, and we all were immensely relieved.

I suffered no setbacks in the hospital, and on dismissal day a week later, my surgeon displayed the results of an echocardiogram taken twenty-four hours before. "Given this result," he proclaimed with a hint of pride, "there's the best possible chance that you will never need another heart operation." Rocky times lay ahead before my recovery was complete, but through them all I was comforted by that blessed thought.

Coming Home

On the plane back to New Mexico—just one week and a day after the operation—I was thumbing through the photo insert in Hillary Rodham Clinton's book *Living History*. One picture broke my heart wide open: the photo of Stevie Wonder playing the song he had written, specifically for her, on the power of forgiveness. There he sat, regal and mellow, making music on a White House grand piano as Hillary inched closer and closer in her chair to capture his words. The picture's caption said she had been "dumbfounded, heartbroken, and outraged" that she had believed her husband's initial denials of involvement with the infamous intern.

As I pondered this photo, I felt the blood coursing through my veins, tingling, warming, gaining momentum. I felt the humming din of the plane engines in my vulnerable chest. The thought that this is the other meaning of the word *heart* was what came to me in the first of a series of emotional outbursts I was to experience in the next twenty-four hours. Stevie Wonder can sing about the power of forgiveness, it struck me, because he has forgiven God for his blindness. Then my tears gushed out. And I can forgive God for my being born with Ebstein's Anomaly. I can let go of my dormant resentment, the anger I've been harboring that I've had to go through all this. I can just let it go! My life is blessed in so many many ways! This was my first tearful release in weeks—and I let it rip.

As it happened, that day—July 24, 2003—was my late father's birthday, the very day on which we would have celebrated his eighty-ninth year if he had not died of a second heart attack in 1957, at the age of forty-two.

The pueblo-style house Bill and I built is not in Santa Fe itself, but twenty minutes outside town, "in the country" in La Paz at Eldorado, and one reason we chose the site was to be able to emote daily over spectacular mountain scenery visible out every window, to savor the 360-degree view.

And there I was, home for two hours, at about 8:00 in the evening, and I still hadn't utterly collapsed after two airplane rides. I went to the window in the master bedroom and gazed out at the dazzling sunset above, the clouds shrouded in pink, purple, rose, gray-blue, and the sheer seventy miles of distance spilling over the green and brown high-desert landscape, the spiritual beauty that drew me here eight years ago… and I burst into tears again. I am so happy to be alive!

I thought. I am so happy for life! I am here living and I just might not have been, because who knew for sure? Yes, I had prepared myself well for the open-heart surgery operation. I had trained myself, if a fear resurfaced, to deliberately fast-forward and imagine a much-loved hike two months in the future. There had been a tiny part of me that wasn't sure I'd make it, and make it I did! I was home again, in my beloved environment, balling away with joy for precious life! Never before do I remember having such a conscious and deep appreciation for the relatively short amount of time we each have here on this planet.

And so I recognized that my sojourn into open-heart territory was ultimately an open heart journey in another sense, a spiritual journey of awakening—to the reality that I am here in this life with a purpose, and have been from the day I was born.

I do not yet know the full spectrum of possibilities to be expressed by that pupose, but it surely includes sharing what I have learned with fellow travelers. If you or someone close to you is facing the prospect of open-heart surgery, I hope this book will provide encouragement, support, and practical guidance as you navigate the road ahead.

PART ONE

What to Do Before
Your Date with
Open-Heart Surgery

CHAPTER ONE

First Steps for the Patient

RECEIVING A DIAGNOSIS that raises the possibility of needing major surgery can be overwhelming, and the prospect of open-heart surgery is particularly frightening. Even if you have weeks or months in front of you for gathering information from libraries or the Internet, the surgery itself looms so large that planning for recovery can seem secondary. But the more you know about exactly what your situation is, about what the procedure entails, and about what to expect afterward, the better able you will be to deal with preoperative fears, the mysteries of your hospital stay, and the process—for some relatively smooth and quick, for others lengthy and difficult—of healing and moving on with your life.

As Dr. Kathleen Blake so rightly points out in the foreword to this book, everyone who faces this experience comes to it with their own strengths and vulnerabilities, both physical and mental. You may recover relatively quickly, or you might have a rockier road to travel. It's my hope that the information in this book, and the guidelines and checklists provided at the back, will be useful to you in any event.

Designate a Caregiver-Advocate

Who will be a full-time set of eyes and ears for you while you are in the hospital? Will your spouse or partner or a close friend be available to oversee your entire stay, follow new developments, take notes for you, ask questions and speak up for you when appropriate? If you anticipate just charging through your surgery experience on your own, think again. If no one close to you is available to be your advocate, seek the support of an internal hospital social worker. It's important that you have a steady ally ready to look out for you at all times. While under the influence of medications and discomfort, you simply won't be your usual, fully in-charge self. The person you choose to help you can also be invaluable in finding answers to such questions as, Can a spouse, partner, or close friend sleep overnight in your hospital room or in the waiting room? What about children—are there age-limit policies on visitation? What insurance issues, like precertification, need to be handled before surgery to qualify you for maximum insurance coverage?

Angela, age forty-six, recently had a heart valve replacement. She put it this way:

You must have an advocate. My husband, Al, and my "nurse" sister were mine. They monitored all the care in the hospital and were certain they were present as doctors made their rounds. They watched over all medications that were administered, confirmed that scheduled tests and procedures were completed, and followed up when necessary. Al later told me about conversations I didn't remember even though I was present. I was surprised to learn that not everyone is fortunate enough to have an advocate with them who is available for the entire hospital recovery.

An advocate who is a relative, spouse or partner, or close friend will also be under stress, and his or her role will extend for weeks or months after you leave the hospital. Chapter 2 is addressed to the caregiver, but it's for you, the patient, as well, for the caregiver supporting you will also need support—including yours.

Get a Second Opinion and Evaluate Your Options

When you receive a diagnosis urging you to consider open-heart surgery, making the decision and selecting a surgeon suddenly become your most urgent priorities. Short of an emergency, no matter how little time you have please get a second opinion, even a third. You will be putting *your life* in this professional's hands. You owe it to yourself to investigate all the risks and benefits, to discuss your alternatives with several close allies, and then—most important of all—to check in with yourself and honor your own gut feeling.

I pursued three opinions. After deliberating with internationally known experts at the Mayo Clinic about my rare congenital valve irregularity and its progressively debilitating effects, I sought referrals from other health professionals and friends. I also went online and found a support group for people with Ebstein's Anomaly (EA), which provided me with firsthand patient reports, including their experiences with the well-known EA specialist surgeon at the Mayo Clinic and with other doctors. Through professional colleagues I was referred to a surgeon at the Cleveland Clinic, another institution highly revered for its outstanding record in cardiac surgery. And last, after faxing the Mayo Clinic's fifteen-page test results to yet another consultant, I spoke with a noted cardiac surgeon at Boston's Brigham & Women's Hospital.

The result? For twenty-five years, the Mayo Clinic in Rochester, Minnesota, had been offering the most commonly recommended surgical procedure for Ebstein's Anomaly, based on the technique of a brilliant surgeon who was now retired. Their current EA specialist had studied at this man's side for ten years, together they had completed five hundred tricuspid valve repairs or replacements for Ebstein's patients, and now the younger man was *the* experienced surgeon for this particular operation. My conversation with the surgeon at the Cleveland Clinic confirmed that he would take an approach similar to that offered at Mayo. But the Brigham & Women's surgeon talked about an entirely new, experimental procedure, a possibility that jarred and confused me. When I reported the Boston approach back to the surgeon and cardiologist at the Mayo Clinic, they replied, "Yes, we know of this procedure, but it's still considered in the experimental stage and we would not recommend it. Even after giving thought to this alternative, we stick by our original proposal for you."

Hearing from a variety of sources about my options was helpful. While it might be upsetting to become temporarily confused while pursuing second opinions, you owe yourself a broad perspective from which to make such an important decision.

Tips on Talking to Doctors

- Get over being shy. Doctors are used to questions.
- Be prepared. Have copies of all test results ready to fax or hand to anyone you're consulting, even though they may want to run their own tests.
- If you're in a managed care health insurance situation, don't be afraid to go beyond the approved list to get an out-of-network second opinion. It will be worth the money even if your insurance won't pay for the visit.
- Ask the surgeon how many procedures he or she, and their team, perform each week. Check if the answer compares favorably with national statistics at www.healthgrades.com. When a team works together

often, its members are likely to be in sync and the operation is apt to go smoothly.

• Ask the surgeon if he or she prefers to have patients on a heart-lung machine during surgery or "off-pump," then weigh the reasons for their preference.

• Write up your list of questions beforehand and ask permission to tape-record the meeting. Ask your caregiver, a good friend, or a family member to accompany you to the consultation. Most physicians will agree to being taped, but for those who won't, remember also to bring a notebook and pen.

In his book *Heal Your Heart: How You Can Prevent or Reverse Heart Disease,* Dr. K. Lance Gould reminds us of the importance of being a knowledgeable patient:

> It is a fundamental axiom that a physician, like anyone else, will deal more carefully with a client who is informed, asking the right questions and expecting rational answers. If the physician is unwilling or unable to engage in a rational discussion of those questions, the client-patient should find another doctor who will.

Tips on Choosing a Hospital

It may seem that since surgeon and hospital go hand in hand, there's nothing to question here. Yet many surgeons perform operations at more than one hospital, and they tend to have strong opinions about them. It might even be the case that you'll be choosing the hospital first, based on what you have learned about its heart surgery department. Hospitals' reputations span from excellent to poor, and everything in between, when it comes to:

- Hygiene protocols
- State-of-the-art technology that can dramatically improve the safety of surgery
- Staffing of cardiac surgery nurses and technicians
- National standard comparison for a heart surgery department

Hospital choice is an area where you can exercise some control. For starters, go to www.healthgrades.com to get an evaluation and ranking for the hospital where the surgeon wants to operate, as well as for the surgeon. Search for additional help on Medicare's www.hospitalcompare.hhs.gov and www.leapfroggroup.org/cp, where data has been offered voluntarily by hospitals.

Another approach is to ask your physicians—surgeon, cardiologist, internist—which hospital they would choose, and why, if *they* were patients. In addition, ask what kind of hospital it is. If it's a teaching hospital, might you be the subject of a study designed to benefit the medical students as much as the patient? Would that be okay with you? Would you prefer a city hospital, where the technology may be more sophisticated and the experience broader, as compared to a smaller private hospital where care may be more personal? In making your decision, consider the following pros and cons of choosing a high-powered out-of-town hospital:

- It may offer the opportunity to choose the "best" surgeon, but it also increases the risk of losing touch with the hospital team once you are home.
- Depending on your insurance coverage, cost may not be a factor, but going out of town could be much more expensive.
- While an institution with a national reputation may offer the latest in technology, a huge medical center can feel like a mill.

Cultivate a Positive Attitude

In the whirlwind of emotions you and your loved ones are experiencing, it may be hard to step away from feeling victimized. After all, you might be in shock, fear, anger, and sorrow all at the same time. Even so, you can *make the choice* to approach your operation positively, and numerous studies have shown that a positive attitude can dramatically influence the outcome.

For decades, respected scientists around the world—working at institutions such as Princeton University, Georgetown University, and the University of Arizona in the United States; McGill University in Cananda; Cambridge University in England; and Okayama University in Japan—have been producing evidence that our thoughts possess an independent energy capable of transforming the nature of our world. In her book *The Field: The Quest for the Secret Force of the Universe,* Lynne McTaggart goes so far as to reference certain experiments by quantum physicists that seem to hint at how our intentions can change physical reality. "Astonishing as it sounds," McTaggart writes, "when we hold a focused thought, it is likely that we are actually making an alteration in the molecular structure of something outside ourselves.... Scientists have now challenged many of the most basic laws of biology and physics." I firmly believe that setting an intention for a positive experience—*believing* you will have a positive outcome—can lead to a speedier, less stressful recovery.

Fortunately, many programs to help people prepare for major surgery have recently sprung up. It is vital to locate such a support, no matter how little time you have before surgery. I was lucky to know about Peggy Huddleston's program, described in her book *Prepare for Surgery, Heal Faster: A Guide of Mind-Body Techniques,* long before I needed it. Huddleston, a graduate of Harvard Divinity School and a psychotherapist in private practice, shows how positive emotions can enhance healing. First published in 1996, her plan consists of her mid-length paperback book and a twenty-minute relaxation CD or tape. The beauty of the program is that if time is short you still can become far more relaxed before surgery—and significantly boost your confidence—simply by listening to the tape twice a day.

Some cardiac surgery patients I've interviewed report that Belleruth Naparstek's visualization and affirmation tapes—

available in the series *A Meditation to Promote a Successful Surgery*—also are very helpful, particularly the one titled *Successful Surgery*. Others I've spoken to have found materials focusing on surgery or relaxation irritating and much preferred listening to music, from Brahms and Mozart to gospel and rock-and-roll.

Whatever your taste, select supportive books, tapes, and CDs to work with in advance of surgery and also at home during recovery. In addition, bring an inspirational and invigorating or soothing supply of music to the hospital to listen to during the surgery (yes, that's possible, and may even have a positive effect on your outcome) and throughout the vulnerable week afterward.

An Exercise for Overcoming Fear and Envisioning Hope
When you're faced with open-heart surgery, it's important to be real with yourself. Toward that end, try working with this brief three-part exercise.

Confront your top ten worries about getting through your operation. Write them down, telling yourself the whole truth. What might some of your worries be?
- How will I *know* I'll make it through the surgery?
- What will be covered by my insurance company and what will I have to pay for?
- What if the anesthesia makes me sick?
- I could develop complications, possibly serious infection.
- Maybe I won't heal correctly.

- Will I get my full stamina and energy back?
- Under any circumstances, I am not ready to die now.

Next, imagine ten things you look forward to after your surgery.
What might you hope for?

- My disease will be corrected!
- My masterful surgeons will return a beautiful quality of life to me!
- I will regain a hundred percent of my strength, and feel better than I have in months, maybe years!
- I will appreciate the gift of life as never before!
- Once again I will walk, run, hike, bike, play tennis!
- I will thrill to a renewed sense of purpose!

Finally, state this claim: I have so much more life to live!

Gather a Community of Friends around You

Short of emergency admittance, no matter how little time you have before open-heart surgery, create a loving support group to surround you. Even though you may feel shy, share your medical challenge with a large circle of friends and family, including colleagues at work and people you know through associations, clubs, organizations, the golf course, your exercise network, book or dinner groups. Extend your reach creatively and you will receive enormous emotional support in return. Many people will ask, "How can I help?" And most of them will have something, no matter how small, to offer.

Consider the types of concrete assistance you and your caregiver will need from others. There's much to attend to before, during, and after a surgical procedure, so match up members of your circle with roles that suit them. Someone will like making phone calls for you; another person will prefer remaining in the background running errands; a third might offer to pray with you over the phone. (Turn to Chapter 4 for more about how to organize a "home team.")

In preparation for the surgery itself, when friends inquire how they can help, ask them to mark their calendars with the day and hour of your operation. Request that they send you loving, healing thoughts and prayers at that very time. One fellow cardiac patient I interviewed told me that before his procedure he had emailed his friends, saying: "Please keep me in your thoughts and prayers (or whatever it is that you do) on Tuesday morning. I can use all the help I can get!"

Consider Listening to Music or Healing Affirmations in the OR

Multiple studies worldwide have shown that even when we are fully anesthetized we never stop hearing what's going on around us, and some studies suggest that we are powerfully influenced by what we hear. This leads many to believe that music or affirmative, healing statements permeating the environment of the operating room itself can directly influence a positive surgical outcome.

If you believe it would be beneficial to you, inform both your surgeon and the anesthesiologist beforehand that you want to listen to music (via earphones connected to a tape or CD player) or would like someone on the surgical team, such as the anesthesiologist or an operating-room cardiac nurse, to read a series of affirmations you have prepared. I printed out my affirmations in big, bold, 16-point type on large, 8-by-11-inch paper and brought two copies with me into the OR, one for the person who would be reading them and a second just for good measure.

Have Your Affairs in Order
While, fortunately, our odds for successful open-heart surgery are higher today than ever before, we need to contemplate the (probably slight) possibility that we will not survive. No matter how well prepared we are for the surgical date, no matter how sure we are that we have chosen the best surgical team, we would do well to put our affairs in order. This means updating your will—or writing one if you haven't done so—reviewing and updating trusts and beneficiaries, and making burial wishes known. It means naming healthcare proxies (people who can make medical decisions if you cannot), appointing someone through a power-of-attorney document to make decisions about finances and property, and writing out clear instructions regarding the removal of life support (a "Living Will"). It's also important to prepare a list of computer passwords, where safety deposit

box keys and the like are to be found, and where important documents, including deeds and insurance policies,
are located.

Additionally, this is a good time to have a frank conversation or two about life and death with someone near
and dear. Because dying is a possibility, albeit remote, consciously acknowledge what the precious gift we call life
means to each of you. These conversations will help affirm
your reality and strengthen the ties that bind you with those
you care most about. You might then compose shared affirmations, formally or informally, to be called upon during
the bumpier moments of the journey ahead.

One caregiving spouse, whose husband had a mitral
valve repair at age fifty-four, told me:

> When my husband went into the hospital, he had
> no will, no living will, nor power of attorney. Be-
> tween the time he entered the hospital and went
> into surgery, all these documents got created and
> signed. It was a tremendous relief for me to know
> clearly what his wishes were in case anything went
> wrong. As it was, he had a complication that made
> things very frightening. I know that having these
> documents before the surgery alleviated what could
> have been overwhelming anxiety. In a strange way,
> having this handled gave me much more confi-
> dence to act with authentic authority on his behalf.
> I can't imagine going through this life-changing

experience without having had these important
documents at hand.

Acknowledge Your Limits

Identify your unique coping style. As far as hearing advance
information, for example, the pendulum swings from patients
who want to be informed about every grizzly medical detail
to those who don't want to know a thing, traversing all variations in between.

Also assess your coping style. Ask yourself what you
need to know to be self-assured before the surgery date, and
the amount of detail. This way, if you are especially anxious,
or if certain mental images will wreak havoc in your dream-
land, you can let health professionals know where you stand
and thus prevent unpleasant encounters with those whose
job it is to help you.

Personally, I fall into the more nervous side of the equa-
tion. I prefaced many conversations with this request: "I
need to let you know that I don't do well hearing about
every medical detail. I will be fully present to respond to
whatever you need me to do, such as how to move my
body, but I ask *not* to hear an in-depth description of any
procedure, particularly while it's going on."

For example, I learned that an angiogram—one of the
tests required before many open-heart surgeries—is an x-ray
examination of the heart and associated blood vessels following the injection of a contrast dye, and for me knowing
only that much was enough. Another heart patient might

have wanted more details about exactly what the procedure involves, but, knowing myself, I chose to end the discussion there, and for me it was empowering to set a boundary that served my needs and temperament. The more I established boundaries with each pre-op or hospital staffer, and combined that with "learning the ropes," the more I increased my self-confidence and reduced my stress about the operation to come.

I recently asked Jodi, a sixty-two-year-old psychotherapist who underwent an aortic valve replacement in August 2005, how much is "too much" to learn in advance about the open-heart surgery experience. This is her reply:

> It's a fine line, how much you can take in beforehand. I actually freaked out by *over*researching, and ended up asking for antidepressants. If people know themselves well, they are generally an accurate gauge of their capacity. It is a good idea to know that depression is a possibility beforehand. It is good to know the procedures that will be performed on you, and about the extensive tubing you will wake up with. Most of all (1) set your own limits and (2) avoid hearing horror stories.

Knowledge *is* empowering, yet being inundated with too much specific information can sometimes be as counterproductive as having too little. The important point is to educate yourself so that you can plan for your surgery and recovery, and at the same time set a threshold regarding the amount of detail that can best help you prepare for it.

CHAPTER TWO

Advice and Support
for Caregivers

*"The ideal advocate is comfortable asking endless
questions and confronting nurses and doctors when
necessary,"* says Ilene Corina, a board member of the
National Patient Safety Foundation.

— *REAL SIMPLE* MAGAZINE, MARCH 2005

WHETHER YOU ARE THE SPOUSE or partner or close
friend of a heart surgery patient, the role of primary caregiver is not an easy one. Before the
operation there's a lot to do, whether you have months or
weeks or even only days to prepare. And there will be new
challenges to cope with during the recovery period

In between, while the surgery itself is taking place, you'll
spend anxious hours in a family waiting area. A hospital staffer
will probably be checking in frequently with updated information: "The patient is now in the OR," "The procedure is going

well," "The patient has been moved to the ICU, the surgeon will speak with you shortly, and soon you will be able to visit for a few minutes..." But those hours are long and stressful, so be sure to ask someone to be *your* companion, to sit with you throughout.

Being an Advocate Before the Surgery

As primary caregiver, you'll have many questions before the operation. It's important to not be intimidated by the shock of what you're dealing with, and to get those questions answered as they come up. Trust your instincts. Carry a notebook and pen with you at all times and take notes. Include the date and any comments or questions that come up during medical consultations with physicians, interns, nurses, or technicians; also record test results as they are reported to you.

Be persistent. It's difficult in a doctor's office or in a bustling and unfamiliar hospital setting to absorb information that comes at you. Request a second explanation if the first doesn't satisfy you. You may need to ask the same or similar questions repeatedly, or even turn to another person on the medical team if your intuition nudges you in that direction.

Here are some examples of the kinds of questions you may have:

- What are the potential side effects of this medication (by mouth, by IV)?
- What, exactly, does that pre-op test or procedure involve?

- How does this hospital's success rate for avoiding infection compare to the national standard? How does the facility rate on www.healthgrades.com?
- What percentage of patients in the care of your hospital's surgical team has suffered a postsurgery stroke?
- What complementary therapies are available—massage, reflexology, acupressure, acupuncture, Reiki, Therapeutic Touch?
- How long will the patient be out of work?
- What about the stairs at home? Should I rent or buy a bed for the first floor?
- Once home, what would tip us off about a need to call 911?

Practicing Assertive Communication

There's a fine line between being a nuisance patient or caregiver, and being a proactive one. But the truth is—whether the focus is on your needs or those of the person you're advocating for—unless you speak up and ask questions, you aren't taking an active enough role, especially in this day and age.

In the June 27, 2005 *Publishers Weekly* cover story on how "health-care consumers" are turning to authors for medical information, writer Natalie Danford laments:

> In 2000, the average patient visit to a physician lasted a scant 18 minutes, according to the U.S.

Department of Health and Human Services.
Less doctor-friendly sources give current dura-
tions as low as five minutes.

In my experience, based on many conversations with
heart patients and their partners and caregivers, doctors seem to fall into two categories. There are those who
will truly listen to you and others who will expect you to
take orders, will have limited sensitivity, and are likely to
become easily irritated when questioned. Beth, one of the
most forthcoming caregivers I interviewed, told me:

> At the first hint that the cardiologist was not an
> ally to us as a couple (he was technically excellent,
> but a terrible communicator and prone to making
> judgments about me based on third-hand infor-
> mation), I wish I'd said we needed a different car-
> diologist. If that weren't possible, I'd have found a
> way to take my husband elsewhere. My intuition
> that this cardiologist disliked me intensely was
> confirmed once I asked our then-family doctor
> for my husband's complete file and saw two letters
> from the cardiologist that really were disrespectful.
> He was totally off the mark about who I am and
> my role as a family member.

There is no excuse for *anyone*—a doctor, medical technician, or hospital staffer—to treat patients or family members

with anything less than full respect, or not to give you the professional time you need. Dr. Eric Rose, chairman and surgeon-in-chief of the Department of Surgery at Columbia University Medical Center, stated in "The Informed Patient," an article printed in the September 9, 2004 issue of the *Wall Street Journal:*

> Arguably, the most important thing is that you have not only a technically competent surgeon but one that you can talk to who knows how to communicate.

Bottom line: if you feel that the physician you and the patient are dealing with is simply not a good match, it may be best to "fire" this person and move on. Pick your battles and educate yourself about your alternatives, but remember to keep your sights set on ensuring the best possible medical partnership.

Providing Support and Encouragement After the Surgery
During the week or so in the hospital after surgery, there are lots of ways the caregiver can fully participate. Above all, dole out good cheer!

In addition, heart patients need to be encouraged to remain active, including lengthening the distance they walk in the hospital corridors, even when walking causes discomfort. They need to be encouraged to cough (to keep the lungs clear) and to continue deep-breathing exercises. It's also very important that they take in plenty of nourishing food and enough liquid. In the event of an initially poor appetite, you can encourage your patient to eat by bringing in familiar homemade dishes or other special treats from the outside.

Once home, the intensity of the primary caregiver's participation ratchets up. The patient, now completely your charge, tires immediately from virtually any activity, a situation that is likely to continue for days and weeks. Frequent rest periods are a necessity, but the recovering patient also needs to build strength by gradually increasing the distance he or she walks every day. Your job is to help find a good balance.

Meanwhile, you'll probably be doing pretty much everything around the house, picking up all the tasks that were previously shared. You'll be the chauffeur for four to six weeks. It's likely that you'll both have trouble sleeping at night because discomfort keeps the patient from finding a tolerable sleeping position, so you may need to get creative about sleeping arrangements. (One couple I know rented a La-Z-Boy–type recliner for the patient to rest and sleep on in the living room, with the caveat that it be used for only a short time after surgery, since sleeping with the head elevated can increase the risk of blood clots in the legs.)

The recovery period is lengthy, and you may face setbacks, however minor. Don't be surprised if you feel annoyed, tired, and sorry for yourself at times. As Audrey, her husband's primary caregiver after quintuple bypass surgery, said, "This kind of caregiving doesn't come naturally, like being a mom did for me. It's not like I had an instinct for this role." If you have children at home, expect the recovery period to be even more complicated, and consider organizing a "home team" (see Chapter 4) to assist and support both your heart patient and yourself!

Caring for Yourself
So what becomes very important? Taking care of *yourself* too. If fatigue and stress threaten to overwhelm you, don't hesitate to ask your doctor for an antianxiety medication so you can ensure quality sleep each night. And from the beginning, *ask for help* from family and friends, especially if you also have children to care for.

Get over being shy. Get over thinking you might be imposing. Some people will turn down a request but most will not. Plan breaks for yourself. Set aside time for a long walk with your dog—or a bike ride, a hike, or an exercise or yoga class—and ask a friend to cover for you while you're out. Make sure you get emotional support as well. If appreciation from your loved one is not forthcoming, by all means ask for it. If he or she cannot give it to you in that moment, call a close friend for some reassurance and perspective. You cannot continue to give without resentment unless you yourself are being taken care of. Reach out to friends, neighbors, even a counselor for short-term support. Caring for yourself—and taking these initiatives—are your responsibility.

My husband Bill was an extraordinary caregiver, filled with patience and endurance that carried us through for many weeks. Somehow I instinctively knew he needed my love and appreciation every day, and no matter how poorly I felt I was still able to let him know how much his efforts meant to me. We were a great team. And once I was able to drive again and feel well enough to stay home on my own, I encouraged him to take blocks of time off for himself. When asked later for thoughts about his caregiving experience, Bill said:

> It was wonderful to receive appreciation from Maggie. She thanked me many times for my attentiveness and care. She encouraged me to be with other people, to take breaks from her needs, to go on a trip. I did! I rode a bike down from the top of Pike's Peak (14,000 feet) in Colorado, a thrill she encouraged. I'm grateful for Maggie and for her reinvigorated health.

"Buddy systems" also can be helpful for both you and the patient in recovery. In addition to talking to the physician about any questions that come up, consider seeking information from former heart patients and caregivers who have "been there." Find a local support group, or tap into a phone or online network (see "Resources" at the back of this book) for more information. And should something disturbing come up, don't hesitate to get medical advice, even if your patient balks.

Monitoring Your Patient's Emotional State

There is often a noticeable difference in how women and men behave during recovery. In my own discussions with patients, women appeared more openly emotional, while most men tended to "task through" their challenges.

In *The Cardiac Recovery Handbook,* Dr. Paul Kligfield, medical director of the Cardiac Health Center at the Weill-Cornell Center of New York-Presbyterian Hospital, and his coauthor offer this message to caregivers:

> As the spouse or close family member of a heart patient, you are in a unique position to observe the emotional changes of your loved one. Unfortunately, you may also bear the brunt of the sadness, bitterness, and anxiety as it arises in your spouse. Your support and help are a crucial component in your spouse's recovery. Numerous studies have shown that mildly depressed patients are more likely to respond to treatment and to recover if they feel loved and supported by family and friends.
>
> Similar studies have also shown that this is not true of people who are severely depressed. They are likely to be unresponsive to your efforts to care for them. They may even be hostile to your care, so you will need outside additional help.

Two final thoughts in this connection. First, in doing research for this book, I heard several reports of temporary personality change. Just as open-heart patients can experience on-and-off bouts of depression (see Chapters 5 and 10), so can they exhibit intermittent out-of-character behaviors causing a normally cheerful person to display persistent grumpiness, lack of cooperation, little or no appreciation. Please don't tolerate this. As the designated caregiver, you deserve steady amounts of copious appreciation and love. So stand up for yourself, and find an empathetic way to communicate your grievances to your loved one.

Second, heed Dr. Kligfield's advice and get extra help if it seems that the person you are caring for is severely or persistently depressed. Begin by asking your medical team, your own doctor, or friends and family for a referral to a mental health professional.

Some Final Words of Encouragement

Even if your heart patient's recovery is swift—and it may well be—there's no straight line to the finish. You may enjoy days of marked improvement when you both breathe a sigh of relief knowing that getting back to "normal" is ahead of you, then hours when recovery seems stalled or even impeded by a setback. It takes a lot of patience, endurance, and trust to keep the healing process on track. Commit to a plan today, then affirm often that one day a year from now you will celebrate the renewal of life and health together.

And remember the old saying about "silver linings." Looking back on her caregiving experience, Beth had this to say:

I now feel a greater sense of competency and mastery in handling things in general, but especially with some of the problems I had to solve while my husband was recuperating. Going through his recovery as a caregiver also encouraged me to be much more physically active. In a way, I had no choice—but instead of seeing taking care of my husband as a chore, I saw it as an opportunity to grow.

CHAPTER THREE

Take an Active Role from the Beginning

ACTIVELY PLANNING FOR your own care will help boost your self-confidence and lessen any fears you may have. And the more you learn in advance, the easier your open-heart journey will be. To get started, identify the strengths you already have. Are you courageous, or resilient? Do you partner well with others? Can you find humor in challenging situations? Drawing on your particular strengths, love yourself and proceed to take an active role each step of the way toward your date with surgery and beyond. For support in initiating specific actions, refer to "Guidelines and Checklists" on pages 171–176.

Learn as Much as You Can about What to Expect
In order to plan ahead for your operation, at the least you'll want to go over the highlights of the hospital's

take-home instruction packet well before your surgery date. If your nerves are frayed, ask your spouse or other designated caregiver-advocate to review it first then give you a summary. In addition to written materials, the patient education departments of many hospitals provide a video portraying what to expect during a hospital stay, which can be very useful in preparing yourself mentally. Your primary caregiver can review it first.

From the very beginning, involve your caregiver—your designated advocate—in every aspect of the proceedings. Let this person in on the details, the worries, the nerve-racking realities you are facing. In turn, let your caregiver tell you about his or her challenges, too, since it's also demanding to be a caregiver. Listen to each other with deliberate consciousness. Ideally, you should each be a sounding board for the other.

Some patients want to know only what they need to know; others want to find out about everything up front. They want to follow the monitors during a heart catheterization. They want to watch and understand the echocardiogram in progress. They want to know the probability of needing a blood transfusion during surgery, and exactly how long it will take for the six-to-eight-inch chest scar to fade away. Ask for the information you think you need.

No matter what level of information will help you cope with the new situation, make every effort to attend the education classes offered at the hospital. (If your surgery is to be performed out of town, request that a copy of available educational videos be mailed to you.) With some early big-picture education, guided by your own gut feeling for how much information you can digest at a time, you'll have a head start in caring for your body and your psyche.

Prepare Advance Questions for the Surgeon and the Anesthesiologist

If you haven't already, you may want to ask your surgeon:

- How exactly do you part the sternum to get to the heart? How long will it take for the incision and the bone to heal?
- Will the anesthesiologist be available to meet with me at least a day before the surgery?
- What are the chances I'll need a blood transfusion? Am I at risk for anemia during my recovery period?
- What are the major potential complications you will be monitoring me for? Infection? Bleeding? Stroke? Reaction to meds?
- Will I be given patient-controlled analgesia (PCA) in an IV, for pain?
- How long do you expect I'll remain in the ICU? How many of my family members will be allowed into the ICU at one time?
- How soon will you get me out of bed? How soon before I can take a shower?
- Will you be recommending I enroll in a cardiac rehabilitation program, and if so, how soon after surgery?

- Is there a former patient of yours who has been through this particular operation and might be willing to receive a phone call from me?

And, if you have the chance, you may want to ask the anesthesiologist:
- In addition to medications, are there specific allergy events I have had that you would like me to expand upon?
- May I tell you what is worrying me most?
- Will you give me drugs for nausea if I become nauseous from the anesthesia?

Make up your own list of questions for the surgeon and the anesthesiologist on what to expect. Bundling your questions and perhaps faxing them on ahead of a consultation is a good way to respect their tight schedules. Not only will it be appreciated, it will also help ensure that you get all the information you're after.

Brush any feelings of intimidation aside and continue to ask *all* your questions. Your advocate can take notes or ask permission to tape the conversations. (A simple "micro" cassette recorder costs about thirty dollars at Radio Shack—an investment that can be worth its weight in gold in terms of reassurance. I remember returning to several key points my surgeon had made during consultations, points that I had not understood or retained at the time.) And don't be shy about telling them your worries and asking for clarification, or asking to hear an explanation repeated and simplified for you a second time.

Befriend the Physician's Assistant

The physician's assistant (PA), can be your lifeline to an on-the-go, sometimes inaccessible surgeon, especially when it comes to those questions that inevitably surface just after you've spoken to the doctor. Keep a list of those, too, to ask the PA.

Having a good relationship with the PA will also make it easier to get answers to additional questions you may have during your recovery. Even though you will be monitored by your regular doctor once home, establishing your surgeon's PA as an ally before the operation paves the way to effective communication with the cardiac team after you have left the hospital.

Check Out Presurgical Procedures and the ICU

Once at the hospital, or even before you get there, you'll be scheduled for several procedures, from straightforward blood tests and X-rays to more sophisticated protocols, like an echocardiogram or an angiogram. Find out beforehand which tests will be required. If you are unfamiliar with any of them, ask the PA about what's involved, and if you need more information than he or she provides, request a contact number for a nurse or medical technician who can talk to you about exactly what to expect.

After your surgery, you will spend a day or two in the intensive care unit (ICU), where you will be monitored closely, especially during the period immediately after the operation. Consider asking to take a quick tour of the facility in advance, if possible. Just as it's reassuring to check out in advance the location for a speech or presentation you're going to give, it's good to have a prior image of the ICU and its staff. Again, the fewer surprises the better. (In my experience, the ICU nurses were among the most caring and dedicated of all those I encountered.)

Be Proactive to Deter Infection
A heart surgeon I know who said she would turn down a job offer at a particular hospital unless its rules for hand-washing were upgraded to a more stringent standard for all medical personnel, accepted the position only after she was promised compliance. This is an important issue nationwide. According to 2002 estimates from the Centers for Disease Control, more than two million hospital patients are struck by infection each year, and while there is no such thing as a perfectly antiseptic environment, experts say that enforcing stricter standards will reduce that number. It behooves you to request—politely, of course—that people who will be touching you first wash their hands with soap and water, or use an alcohol-based hand sanitizer. Insist on it.

Get Contact Information and Plan for Follow-up Care
Many patients experience a major sense of "disconnect" from the hospital medical team once they are released and land at home. I did, and I've spoken with several heart surgery patients who concur. The surgeon, other physicians, and overworked residents and nurses are focused on getting

the patient *through* the surgery to approximately one week beyond. Since managing a lengthy period of homecare is not their job, the preparation they will give you for the early stages of recovery may very from excellent to poor. Although they are familiar with their patients' take-home literature, and PAs and nurses may give out additional, more personalized instructions that are very helpful, you need to know more than just that "you will have good days and bad days."

Ask the PA or discharge cardiac nurse to sit down with you, tell you what to *really* expect (particularly in the first two or three weeks), and give you any practical advice they can about coping with the challenges ahead—physical *and* psychological. Ask whom you can contact for support during the first few weeks of your recovery, *especially* if you've had your surgery far from home. This includes a contact to call with concerns at night and on weekends. Even though you anticipate being monitored by your local physician, the PA or the assigned cardiology nurse should literally hand you a phone number or two. As the ad says, *Don't leave home [the hospital] without it!* Giving you this reality-check briefing should be part of the PA's job description, so don't be shy about asking for it.

The experience of coming home after major surgery can be compared with bringing home your first baby, for no matter how much research you've done, you are now wearily and dizzyingly on your own, and it's important to be able to quickly contact the appropriate person to help you solve any problems that arise.

If you are having your operation locally, you will likely be visiting your surgeon within the first two weeks, and you may have other initial follow-ups, by phone or in person, with the PA or cardiology nurse. If you have traveled a distance to have your surgery performed, take home a clear directive regarding who to consult, and when. When I left the Mayo Clinic, following my open-heart surgery repair, I was instructed to visit my local physician within the next seven to ten days. As it turned out, my primary physician was on vacation when I returned home, and so I was seen by a substitute internist in the same practice. For the kinds of heart-related questions I had about my fatigue, sleep issues, depression, and pain medication mix, an experienced cardiology nurse might have been the more suitable recommendation. Especially before leaving a distant hospital, ask the surgeon's PA to help you coordinate follow-up care.

Discuss the Issue of Pain Management
Make it a priority to discuss how you'll manage postoperative pain and discomfort, both during the hospital stay and once you are home. How does your doctor plan to manage your pain in the ICU and afterward? Injections? Pills? Will you automatically be given medication for nausea or will you have to ask for it? Will you be offered a patient-controlled IV? How long is pain likely to last?

In the hospital, you'll have an array of experienced medical personnel attending you. Meds for just about anything (nausea, sleeping challenges, constipation) are available at the touch of the nurse call button. Once home, however, *you* will be making all the immediate decisions. You are in charge of deciding what your level of pain tolerance is, how much medication to take and when, and the rate at which to taper off any painkillers or meds you've been given for other kinds of discomfort. We each have our individual pain thresholds and tolerances, so initiating a preliminary conversation on the choices for pain management at home will serve you well. While many people are justifiably wary of pain medications, you don't want to let your pain get out of control. Keeping in touch with your medical advisors and listening to your own body will help you strike a balance.

Seek Practical Advice about Things to Watch Out for

It is essential to partner beforehand with everyone on your medical team. Jim, a tall, sturdy man who at age seventy-two had recently undergone a mitral valve repair, told me he wished he'd been given some "bedside physics" instructions before going into the hospital. What he was talking about is this. You're used to using the full range of motion of your arms to get in and out of bed, and also to turn while you're lying down, but after surgery the tissue in your chest will be very sore. It needs time to heal, and instinctively we accommodate by inventing other ways to move our bodies (I learned to use my elbows only). Other people have been in this situation before, however, so it's not necessary to root around for solutions. Experienced nurses may be able to give you some presurgery movement lessons that will help avoid several weeks of roving shoulder and back aches in bed. Inquire about this beforehand, then practice any suggested maneuvers, especially for getting in and out of bed, before you have the surgery.

Learn, and take responsibility for, as much as you can absorb about the physiological and psychological challenges you may encounter once you are home. When you and your primary caregiver review the highlights of the take-home instruction packet with the PA, inquire about common issues to specifically watch out for. Ask about fatigue and depression—what to expect and how to manage it. Review a list of your prescribed medications, over-the-counter remedies, vitamins, herbal supplements, and even any illegal drugs. (Most likely you will have been advised to eliminate some of them a week or two before the surgery date.) And don't forget to ask which signs should prompt you to call your doctor from home immediately.

Investigate Complementary Healing Remedies and Therapies
There is a reason why complementary care centers are springing up in hospitals all across America. To quote from *Healing from the Heart,* by heart surgeon Mehmet Oz, who works at the Columbia Presbyterian Medical Center in New York City:

> I sometimes tell my skeptical peers that it's not so much whether this or that therapy has clearly proven clinical value, but that Americans are voting

for complementary medicine with their dollars. According to a recent joint study by Boston's Beth Israel Hospital and Harvard Medical School, Americans spend about $14 billion a year on these therapies and their products, such as vitamins and herbal remedies....Moreover, investigators estimate that one out of three Americans resorts to these therapies, with seven out of ten users *never* telling their personal physician about these consultations or treatments.

For example, if you're unfamiliar with the use of acupuncture to reinvigorate the immune system after surgery, gather information from friends who have experienced positive outcomes. You might want to line up a massage therapist for once you are home. Herbal remedies can be helpful, but many "natural" products interact with prescription medications, so be sure to consult your primary physician about any herbals you are considering taking. Investigate and welcome the existence of both Western medical and complementary healing approaches. Don't fall into the either/or trap. Use the best healing approaches of both. (See "Resources," on pages 181–184, for suggested reading.)

You might also consider requesting Therapeutic Touch (TT) during the forty-eight hours surrounding your operation. According to Peggy Huddleston, more than 50,000 nurses have been trained to offer this calming, healing treatment that can be performed if you simply know in advance to request it, and chances are that you can locate a practitioner within the hospital. Even if the nurse you've contacted is not part of your immediate surgical team, she or he will do their utmost to be there with you when you are about to enter the OR, in the ICU, and once again back in your hospital room. Without touching your body, the TT practitioner influences the energy field around you with gentle hand motions. The experience can be wonderfully soothing, especially within the context of a bustling, high-tech hospital setting.

Practice Good Self-Care
Taking an active role from the beginning also calls for practicing good self-care. You need your sleep, you need a nourishing diet, you need time-outs. Plan times to relax on your own. Arrange for exercise, even if it's just walking three times around the block. Anything you can do to maximize your health and well-being ahead of time will stand you in good stead.

CHAPTER FOUR

Organize a Home Team

Perhaps the shortest and most powerful
prayer in human language is Help.

—FATHER THOMAS KEATING, IN
THE BOOK OF AWAKENING BY MARK NEPO

EVEN IF YOU HAVE VERY LITTLE TIME before your heart surgery, organize a home team before you go in. If you are just home from the hospital, it's still not too late. Make a list of family and friends (but not your primary caregiver) who would be glad—if not honored—to be called to help out. From among them, pick a leader to contact the others about the tasks ahead, with the goal of setting up a schedule of assignments they would be willing to take on during your first three or four weeks back home.

A Friend? Why Not Your Primary Caregiver?

Whoever your primary caregiver will be—your spouse, your partner, a friend, another family member—once you are home and recovering, the scenario will change. Suddenly that individual, your close personal ally, has the extended responsibility for all regular household tasks plus new ones: nursing aid, transportation, medical and social plan coordination. Your primary caregiver, now "on" 24/7, needs assistance, too. This is why you line up a home team to pitch in.

Of course, your caregiver will also need continuing acknowledgment, appreciation, and love from you. Plan to regularly express your gratitude. Find out how he or she is feeling—every day. Though sometimes you won't feel like it, remember to do your best to smile and show you care!

Five Basic Ways the Team Can Help

1. Preparing dinner nightly. Some friends will want to prepare a home-cooked meal for both patient and caregiver, while others might prefer to deliver heart-healthy take-out food. Since the reality of landing back home means the primary caregiver is focused on you so much of the time, he or she will appreciate a sit-down break for something good to eat, especially at dinnertime.

2. Providing emotional support and practical advice. During the many hours and days of convalescence, neither patient nor primary caregiver wants to feel isolated at home.

So think about setting up some buddy systems in advance. Is there a friend, or a friend of a friend, who has been though open-heart surgery and is willing to talk about their experience, or even to check in with you regularly? Is there a support group in your area whose members could be available by phone to give practical advice? Many smaller questions can be answered in this way, but keep in mind that substantial recovery questions require a phone call to your designated medical professional. You and your caregiver should also plan regular private time with best friends, in person or by phone, to freely let your hair down and tell it like it is!

3. Running errands. Who—friend or neighbor—would be willing to be counted on to run to the pharmacy? To deposit or pick up laundry or dry cleaning? To shop for staples at the supermarket? To buy a box of thank-you notes? Ask your team leader to recruit a list of volunteers beforehand.

4. Housekeeping. In the hospital take-home instructions you receive, there will be very specific physical directives that must be honored while the sternum (breastbone) is healing. You are not to lift more than five to ten pounds for six weeks. In addition, you are to avoid both pushing and pulling activities with your arms and also heavy one-armed lifting for three months. This eliminates hauling groceries, carrying a toddler, vacuuming, shoveling snow, mowing the lawn, raking leaves; even wiping a kitchen counter with a sponge can be challenging in the first couple of weeks. So plan to call on others for help with regular housekeeping chores for at least four to six weeks, or consider hiring a professional house cleaner for that period.

5. Chauffeuring. An open-heart surgery patient may not resume driving for four to six weeks, until the sternum is fully healed, but can ride in a car as soon as they're home— to a medical appointment, to the store, to eat out. (See page 98 for the latest guidelines on airbags and restraints, and other protective devices.) All these outings add up to a lot of driving for the primary caregiver, however, so line up chauffeur volunteers to give your caregiver a break.

Overcoming Resistance to Asking for Help

When I was encouraged to plan ahead in this way, I resisted at first. Push my "ask for help" button and I tend to recoil. But I was eventually persuaded and began by asking my friend Paula to arrange for other friends to bring in dinner for the first two weeks of my convalescence. The point is, it's tough enough to envision getting through the open–heart operation itself, and while you're facing that challenge it's daunting to simultaneously imagine being laid up for weeks. But you must prepare for a four-to-eight-week recovery period during which you won't be up to much. If you have never experienced major surgery, you can't viscerally envision this state of being; besides, you are too busy preparing for the upcoming surgery. So please, call on a close friend in advance, one for whom organizing a group of caring people would be a satisfying way to help, and might even be fun. (The initial request script might go something like this: Would you be free in the two to four weeks after Toby's operation to (1) stop by the home and take care of a housekeeping detail or run an errand, or (2) visit and chat every so often for a few minutes, or (3) bring something over for dinner?)

Arrange for Psychological and Spiritual Support

It's important for both you and your caregiver-advocate to arrange for psychological and spiritual support before, during, and after the operation from people who will be willing to check in on you regularly about your state of mind and soul. They might include a close friend or sibling; a psychotherapist, counselor, or coach; your pastor, your rabbi, or another spiritual practitioner.

Ask the designated person (or two) to call on a regular basis, to ask questions, to see how you both are faring psychologically and spiritually. If you are struggling, if you seem in a fog, if something is just plain "off," that person will catch it and pitch in to help with next steps, which might include longer conversations, counseling with a qualified coach or mental health professional, or prayer or healing circle sessions.

Designate a Follow-up Communicator

The day of, or the day after, surgery, everyone connected to your inner circle will want to hear *something*. They will want to be assured you've made it through and are doing well. Anticipate the different levels of communication appropriate for family and friends. Compile a list of phone numbers or prepare email groupings, then designate one individual to be the first-line communicator. If this person is your primary caregiver, he or she could delegate a portion of the task to someone else; perhaps your caregiver will want to make some phone calls directly while another family member or friend sends daily group emails. Spread the "being in touch" around. Involving those closest to you in this process will help them feel they are contributing proactively even before you're out of the hospital.

Prepare Your Home Environment

If there's time beforehand, walk around your home slowly and try to imagine how you can make that environment more functional for your recovery. While climbing stairs usually isn't discouraged after open-heart surgery, if your bedroom is on the second floor it could be more desirable during the first few weeks for you to take your rest in a main-floor room. Are there items in the kitchen or dining area that require reaching up high? To avoid reaching your arms up for anything heavy consider temporarily rearranging some favorite foods, cans, bottles. And what's in the freezer? If there's time, cook some meals ahead and freeze them for later, and stock up on preferred grocery and toiletry items.

Your environment can be an affirming space for you during your recovery if it is practical and cozy. After all, you will be spending many hours, days, and weeks there. A little forethought and some temporary changes can make a big difference. In which rooms will you be most comfortable? Which window will you want to gaze out of this time of year? Where will your meds and your med chart be? Where will you perform your first month's chest-strengthening exercises? Where will you take your daily walks?

Hope for a Swift Recovery, Plan for a Longer One

There is no magical amount of time you can count on as a "number of weeks" measurement for recovery from an open-heart operation. Going into surgery, we are each unique beings with our own histories and proclivities. We intend to heal quickly. We may in fact intend, as I did, to heal in a specific number of weeks. (I had it *scripted* that I would mend in only three weeks. I didn't.) Definitely ask beforehand what the expected recovery period is—*in general*. But remember that the answer your surgeon gives you is just an average, and that recovery takes more or less time for each person.

Finally, with your home team in place, plan to reach out for help whenever you need it. And be sure to express and discuss your feelings with people who are close to you, as well as others who have been through similar experiences. Open-heart surgery is a big challenge, and both you and your caregiver will benefit if you allow others to help you meet it.

CHAPTER FIVE

The Challenges You May Face

RESTING LATE ONE AFTERNOON a few weeks after my homecoming, droopy and irritable about the realities of open-heart convalescence, I began to itemize in my mind the things I might have investigated in advance. True, I had established some excellent links to professional specialists. But I hadn't asked questions about *recovery*. That weary day I acknowledged how little I had known about the challenges now facing me. Had I been told to be on the lookout for conditions like serious constipation, excessive fatigue, and symptoms of depression, I would have acted sooner to get advice about nipping those rascals in the bud.

This chapter addresses a number of issues to know about beforehand so you can better plan your recovery from open-heart surgery. These observations are drawn from my own experience plus perspectives from dozens of open-heart patients I've interviewed. They are intended not to raise alarm but only to prepare you for what otherwise might be unexpected. (This is a partial list only. I welcome feedback from you, the reader, so that I may add your insights and suggestions to a future edition of this book.)

Every *Body* Is One of a Kind

Early on, discuss your particular uniqueness—highlights about *you* physiologically—with your surgeon, your anesthesiologist, and the PA. Since these medical professionals are focused only on getting you through your specific surgery, you can't count on them zeroing in on the sideline details of the medical questionnaire you so carefully completed. It may be in the doctor's folder, but chances are that it won't be consulted again. Everyone is just *so busy.* What with computers, incessant email, fax machines, and ubiquitous cell phones, just plain living has sped up to such a degree that many of us are running faster and harder than ever before, and nowhere is this more evident than in a hospital setting.

Personnel at any well-run hospital are indeed going to ask you repeatedly to spell your name, reiterate your date of birth, and recap the medications you are allergic to. Be concerned if they do not. But you must also educate them about your particular history and concerns: you must be proactive whenever those concerns need to be heard. For example, for me a chronic pain can arise below my left shoulder blade if I'm lying flat on my back for more than a few minutes. Once I tell a medical technician about this, we can negotiate a minimum amount of time I will need to remain in that position—or maybe lying on my side for a given test could work just as well. You need to be ready to speak up and let anyone on your medical team know about such issues at the appropriate time.

Allergic Reactions, Medication Side Effects, and Drug Interactions

The possibility of an allergic reaction to any new anesthesia, anesthesia combination, or pain medication is always present. You don't get a trial run. Since the anesthesiologist has a potpourri of wonder drugs to choose from, the more you present your previous allergic reactions (not just to medications and foods, but are you allergic to bee stings?) the better equipped the anesthesiologist will be to prepare your mixtures—during both your surgery and the hospital days that follow.

The potential for medications not mixing well with one another also exists. You and your caregiver will do well to discuss with the medical team every med you are given at any point: What possible side effects or risks are associated with both the medication and its interaction with the other meds and supplements you are currently taking? (For example, nausea can be a side effect of anesthesia and pain meds for which adjustments are available.) What are the alternatives? How long is it absolutely necessary to remain on a particular regimen? Participate as fully as possible in decisions about everything you agree to feed your body.

Expect Limitations during Recovery

The news that you have coronary artery disease, or a heart valve that needs repair, often comes suddenly, and if you've considered yourself "healthy" up until that pronouncement, chances are you'll assume you'll have a straightforward recovery. But even if you are blessed with a relatively short convalescence, the weeks after surgery will be stressful. Anticipating limitations, accepting them, and adapting to them are all part of taking a proactive role in your return to full health.

Resist Isolation

Once you're home, there you are, every day, attending to your number one job: healing well from open-heart surgery. You are getting stronger. You are adjusting to life's new challenges and requirements. Your goal is to enjoy a new, healthier quality of life in the future. But this process takes time—extended time. Your energy level does not improve overnight, like the beautiful flash of a sudden shooting star in the night sky. You will most likely spend long hours at home, day after day. It may seem like the world is going on without you, which may make you feel isolated.

This is the time to find other open-heart surgery survivors and their caregivers to talk to. Swap stories, share information, hear what other families have gone through. Just knowing that you are not alone as you go through your rehabilitation can lift the veil of isolation. There can be a tendency to hold one's surgery and recovery experiences too privately, but not reaching out to others will only deprive you of receiving compassionate support. If you are feeling isolated, do yourself a favor: reach out to friends and family, and look for a heart surgery support group locally or online.

Be Alert to Signs of Infection and Other Complications

Infection is a possibility worth discussing with your surgeon. Question your surgeon about the medical guidelines to be followed for antibiotic administration before and after surgery to prevent infection. Care of your wound will be monitored during your hospital stay, but once you're home it's very important to honor the take-home instructions you'll be given. Occasionally, recovering patients come down with an infected incision or a systemic infection. The several instruction packets I've seen tell the patient to immediately report fever above 100.4 degrees Fahrenheit (38 degrees Celsius), for instance, or a low-grade fever lasting more than two or three days. Once home, yes, you have survived the risk of infection in the hospital. Now it's imperative to keep up the vigilance on your own.

In addition, since the immune system is compromised from the shock of open-heart surgery, it's wise to stay away from crowds and any individual who has a cold or flu. Immediately following surgery we are simply more susceptible to bacteria and viruses.

One of my setbacks involved the appearance of a low-grade fever and lack of appetite combined with increasing weakness. I figured it must be some virus. Then, during an eight-week cardiac checkup that included an echocardiogram, pericarditis—an inflammation of the membranous sac that surrounds the heart—was identified. I was given an anti-inflammatory drug and within two weeks felt much better. So, again, listen to your own body and err on the side of caution: don't hesitate to phone your designated medical liaison to alert them to anything that feels like a big step backward.

Keep an Eye Out for Symptoms of Depression

Especially with emergency surgery, when there is no time to plan *anything*, acknowledging the potential for post-operative anxiety and depression is important, if not critical. An article by G. Drees and colleagues, titled "Psychological Care Should Be Offered After Open-heart Surgery" and appearing in the August 30, 2004 issue of *Cardiovascular Week*, states:

> Since it is essential to see cardiological rehabilitation following surgical procedures such as coronary bypass surgery, valve surgery, implantation of a cardiac pacemaker or defibrillators also under the aspect of illness management and life-style modification, rehabilitation should not exclusively focus on the physical problems but also take account of the psychological problems of patients.

Even if you are electing open-heart surgery and have time, as I did, to plan ahead, understand that according to multiple studies 30 to 40 percent of open-heart patients experience depression once they are home and recovering. This makes sense, really, because having to undergo open-heart surgery is a trauma to begin with. Therefore be on the lookout for signs of depression, so that you can seek help right away. Common signs of depression include any combination of the following:

- Deep self-doubt
- Difficulties thinking and concentrating
- Sleep and appetite disturbances
- Crying, especially spontaneous spells
- No interest in normally stimulating activities
- Withdrawal from family and friends
- Feelings of hopelessness
- Thoughts of death or suicide

If you or your caregiver suspect you may be mildly depressed, don't turn your back on this hunch. Give yourself permission to discuss your feelings with your primary care physician or cardiologist immediately. Find out how to get short-term counseling with someone who has worked with cardiac patients and is therefore familiar with the medications you are taking. This therapist might be a social worker, a clinical psychologist, or a psychiatrist. In recent years, fortunately, there are new antidepressants on the market that seem generally safe for heart patients. Choose a therapist who is familiar with the newest drugs and has solid experience with drug dosing and documented side effects.

Cognitive Issues

After open-heart surgery, some individuals complain of memory loss, difficulty concentrating, losing their train of thought, forgetting people's names or what they've just read—all similar to the mild cognitive impairment we complain of as we get older. To some extent these issues are common in any patient recovering from major surgery. An open-heart operation, however, presents an additional likely cause—time spent on the heart-lung machine—though that hasn't been proven, and fortunately "post-pump syndrome" seems to be on the decline (see pages 149–151). When cognitive issues arise early on, the symptoms are usually temporary. Patients are routinely reassured that their mental faculties will return, and happily this is generally the case. Better to know in advance that cognitive challenges are a possibility, and to be reassured that they too shall pass.

Bob—who at eighty-one had had both mitral and tricuspid valves repaired, plus one bypass, and who was playing tennis again three months after surgery—had this to say:

> I decided in December to schedule surgery January 8, and for the rest of that month I was out of it. My brain shut off in January, and I worried it wouldn't come back on. Then in February it came on with a rush!

While waiting for your own memory to return to its former reliability, you can compensate and help retrain your brain by taking notes and making lists.

Sleep
Sleeping will be a challenge for a while, and the challenge comes in various guises. One patient friend remarked, "If I'd known I'd have to sleep on my back for two months, I might never have had this operation!" But sleeping on one's side can be a problem as well, either because it's too painful initially (spreading the sternum during surgery puts pressure on one's back and shoulders) or because it brings on back and shoulder discomfort later in the night. To help yourself sleep through the night, you may need to limit daytime napping (while still spending time at rest) or resort to the sleeping aid you may have resisted adding to your multi-pill regimen. Some experimentation and patience will probably be necessary before you figure out what works best for you.

Narcotic Pain Medications and Constipation
Here's a word of advice, again from Angela:

> Understand how to care for your bowels—it took me several weeks to get this regulated, including one near emergency. Given no information, I had to make many calls to doctors and dieticians.

Did you know that when we are on any kind of a narcotic, serious constipation is the usual companion? I did not know this, and surely many of us are ignorant if we haven't had previous experience with prescription pain medication. Since you will likely be given narcotic meds during and after your operation—morphine, its variations, or whatever—discuss a constipation relief plan in advance. Arrange to have plenty of fiber, fruits, bran cereals, and whole grains on hand for your return home. Ask about stool softeners or other relief choices before leaving the hospital. For the duration of time you choose to continue on narcotics such as Percocet, constipation may be an issue. If it becomes persistent, don't hesitate to call someone on your follow-up medical team for help.

Driving and Lifting Restrictions

Although you will not be able to resume driving for four to six weeks, the most recent Mayo Clinic guidelines advise that you need not be confined to the back seat. The use of a commonly available restraint such as a shoulder harness provides you with the best protection against injury whenever you sit in a car. (It was once thought that since a shoulder harness might concentrate the force of an impact in a small area, it might represent a particular danger to someone whose chest is still healing. But now, it's believed, the protection shoulder restraints offer against *other* kinds of injuries seems to far outweigh that risk. Front-seat airbags were once another cause for concern, but since they deploy over the entire chest, current thinking is that they represent less risk in relation to their benefits, although you might want to slide a front-passenger seat back a little to allow the airbag to slow a bit before encountering the chest.)

With regard to lifting, you are to avoid activities that require pulling, pushing, or picking up more than five or ten pounds, for six weeks. I remember testing myself early on by using my right hand to wipe a countertop. Attempting this was *completely* undesirable my first week home. Then a couple of strokes with a sponge would do me in during the second week. But by the third or fourth week I could more or less bear down lightly on the countertop and wipe it for five or six strokes before having to stop to honor the healing of my tender chest muscles. In my passion to get life activities "back to normal," I would overdo it and then regret having pushed myself harder than was wise. So my advice is to go slow and back off whenever your body tells you you're overdoing it.

Anemia

In addition to the narcotic-meds-and-constipation roller-coaster during the weeks following open-heart surgery, there is a significant potential for anemia that doesn't resolve on its own. I have learned that some heart patients are routinely equipped with iron supplements (ferrous gluconate) when they leave the hospital. Others are not (I was among them), because iron may cause either nausea or constipation and, as my very experienced PA at the Mayo Clinic later explained, "The body is uniquely designed to build back the hemoglobin on its own." After a respectable two weeks back home, I hit a downward spiral that was later to be diagnosed as anemia. I felt weaker by the day, rather than better, and couldn't understand why. Suspicious, I insisted on a blood count. The lab report took longer than usual to reach my primary care physician. Then more time elapsed. Finally, it became crystal clear that I was anemic, and that the best choice was to intervene with an iron supplement rather than wait to let my body return on its own to its usual blood count level.

Cardiac Rehabilitation

Prepare for the common physical and psychological challenges of the first four to six weeks of recovery. Please *give yourself permission* to allow for them! Full recovery may take more weeks than you ever imagined. In the meantime, systematically increase your walking every day, to the point where you can visualize and look forward to the strength retraining and aerobic stamina offered in a good cardiac rehabilitation program. Once your doctor finally approves you for cardiac rehab, you will discover what may be a new experience or the reawakening of an old pleasure—going to the gym!

PART TWO

Planning for Your
Hospital Stay

CHAPTER SIX

The Hospital Experience
for First-Timers

IF YOU'VE NEVER BEFORE SPENT time in a hospital, think of your stay as traveling to a new high-tech environment where caring nurses, technicians, physicians, and surgeons have ever-improving control over surgical outcomes. In other words, take the high road. Just as you have thoroughly discussed the benefits and risks of your open-heart operation with your cardiologist, surgeon, and others involved in your decision, you and your caregiver-advocate will gain precious new confidence by taking time to learn the hospital ropes beforehand.

An Overview

As your surgery date approaches and you proceed through your preoperative consultations and tests, you will observe that everyone at the hospital is focused on the specific job they have to do. It's all for your health and well-being, of course, but it's a busy place, and, feeling more vulnerable than usual, you may seem to be caught in a whirlwind. Expect to be ushered from one test to another, from blood draws to X-rays to electrocardiograms, all preparing you for your entrance into the OR. Eventually you'll be following your surgeon's specific "night before" instructions. Then, after surgery, caring nurses will greet you when you wake up in the ICU and again in your hospital room. Most important, keep asking for explanations or procedural clarifications as you need to. If you're not sure what's going on, ask. If you're anxious, you can request a sedative. If you're uncomfortable, physically or mentally, let someone know. You have a right to be involved every step of the way.

Hospital Procedures and Regulations
Whether large or small, local or distant, every hospital has its own identity, set of protocols, financial arrangements, and bureaucratic systems in place. Visit the hospital ahead of your surgery, if possible. Ask lots of questions and note answers. As you meet the nurses and others responsible for taking you through tests and procedures, *be friendly;* even though you are preoccupied with your medical challenges, take the time to remember names as well as professional designations, and relate with a human touch. This will be appreciated and may make all the difference in the attention you receive in return. You are on a mission to educate yourself, and a befriended nurse's perspective can be invaluable.

Once you've become aquainted with your new allies, you're ready to get straight answers to questions like, How does this work here? Are there regulations I specifically need to be aware of?

As a first-timer in the hospital, you may feel clueless about what needs asking. Begin with a list of everything you think it will take to make you feel less anxious and more comfortable. For example, some hospitals won't routinely allow families to visit a patient while in the ICU, but the rules may be flexible. Raise this and other questions that touch on concerns of importance to you. Many hospitals have patient advocates available to help new admissions navigate the system. All you need to do is ask.

Packing Tips
What *not* to bring or wear to the hospital:
- Leave valuables—including jewelry, credit cards, and large sums of money—at home.
- Consider leaving even your wedding ring at home. You will be asked to remove it for the operation anyway. The same holds true for body-piercing ornaments.
- Remove pigmented nail polish so the coloring of finger and toe tips can be closely observed.

What *to* bring to the hospital:
- Minimal extra clothing: clean underwear, a robe, and slippers with rubber soles that will keep you from slipping on polished floors. This is all you'll need

other than loose clothes (consider a front-buttoning garment rather than one that slips over your head) for your return home.

- An updated list of your medications: all prescription drugs (with dosage and frequency), over-the-counter medicines, vitamins, minerals, herbal supplements, and any illegal drugs.
- Important paperwork: your power of attorney for health care and a "living will" spelling out clear instructions about removing you from life support.
- A list of your allergies, not just to medications but also nonpharmaceutical allergies like bee stings or shellfish.
- A list of recent lab tests, X-rays, and other relevant details of your medical history.
- A journal for keeping a medical log.

What you could bring to make your stay more comfortable:
- Audio, MP3, or CD/tape player, and fresh batteries.
- Relaxing music, magazines, books, crossword puzzles.
- Cases for eyeglasses, contact lenses, dentures, hearing aids.
- Cell phone, if permitted (otherwise invest in a long-distance phone card).
- Hairdryer, electric shaver.
- Telephone numbers of family and friends.
- Pillow marked with your name.
- Toiletries, favorite personal hygiene items, makeup.
- Eye mask or earplugs.

Your caregiver's list might include:
- An extra pad or pen.
- Calendar with contact info for family and friends.
- Micro cassette recorder for taping physician meetings.
- Water bottle and healthy snacks.
- A day's worth of personal medication.
- Cell phone or long-distance calling card.
- Reading material, audio, MP3, or CD player.
- Neck pillow.
- Personal hygiene items.
- An extra bag for patient's last-minute items, take-home packets, cards, gifts, and so forth.

Just Before You Go

Plan to leave your household in order. But if there's not much time, at least try to pay last-minute bills that may come due during your absence. Hopefully your "home team" is in place, and child and pet care is now arranged. If you develop a sore throat, a cold, or a fever at the last minute, be sure to check with your surgeon's office immediately. You might have to postpone the surgery.

If all goes well, you'll now need to follow your surgeon's "night before" instructions. You will be told to not eat or drink anything after midnight the night before surgery. Probably you will be given a special antibacterial soap to shower with the night before you leave for the hospital. Be sure to wash your hair as well—it may be a few days before you have that pleasure again!

CHAPTER SEVEN

From the ICU
to the Journey Home

ONCE YOUR SURGERY IS COMPLETED, you'll be transferred to the intensive care unit for the first stage of your recovery. Usually, family may visit the heart patient in the ICU briefly, yet you may not remember seeing them. Most of us don't recall any of our experience in the ICU, and that's a good thing. Most likely you will be spending several hours drifting in and out of sleep while various tubes and monitors assist with your bodily functions and provide continuous data (vital signs, blood pressure, heart rate and rhythm) to the nurses and doctors charged with guiding this stage of recovery of the heart and your overall physical state.

A day after my own surgery, finally waking up in my hospital room, I was ecstatic. I had made it through! I still had equipment protruding from me—drainage tubes out my chest, an IV in my hand, a heart monitor attached to a bow around my neck—but I had *made* it and these accompaniments were just details. Whatever pain medication I was on at that juncture was obviously working. My smiling family members were there when I awoke. Here I was, alive and grinning back at them.

I knew that challenges lay ahead, beginning with those I'd encounter during my week in the hospital, but at that moment life was good!

Living on Hospital Time

It didn't take me long to grasp that there is no rest in the hospital after an open-heart operation. In addition to coping with all the paraphernalia you sport in bed that challenges a decent sleeping position, you might be awakened at 1:00 a.m. for meds after sleeping only a few hours, and again at 3:00 a.m. by a tech drawing your blood for round-the-clock blood chemistry monitoring. Not to mention that the nurse will be in regularly to take your temperature, check your blood pressure, and remind you to cough into a plastic device (to prevent lung complications). Your fluid intake, urine output, and weight will be measured daily, and because early movement is critical for rapid recovery, you will be encouraged to lengthen the time you spend out of bed and the distance you walk along the hospital corridors each day. So best to simply prepare yourself for not getting the quality of sleep you're used to. Your healthcare team will recommend frequent rest periods instead, and it will help to listen to their advice.

Getting Moving Again

The first day or two in your hospital room will feel more challenging than day three and day four and so on. Your sense of fragility and disorientation will lessen as you feel more yourself and begin to move around. I was allowed to take my first shower the second day up, and it was bliss—never mind that this mere ten minutes of chaperoned activity wiped me out and I succumbed to a two-hour nap afterward. Your hospital team will provide you with relevant guidelines, but others also exist online (the Cleveland Clinic's is highly recommended) that will help you anticipate the kinds of activities you will be up to day by day for the week you are in the hospital after your surgery. As that week wears on, tubes come out, monitors get disconnected, your activity increases, and healthcare team supervision becomes less intense.

Accepting Pain Relief

People have different levels of pain tolerance. What registers as severe discomfort for some may be regarded as minor discomfort by others. We ourselves are the best judges of how we feel. In my opinion, it's important not to play Superman or Superwoman and tough it out without any pain relief medication at all. By accepting a prescribed dosage of narcotic pain medication on a regular schedule, at least in the beginning, you may avoid getting into trouble later if you suddenly and desperately need additional relief. Both common sense and current opinion about best practice in this regard tell us we won't get hooked on a narcotic med within a short period of time. So don't be afraid to opt for a decent level of comfort or to ask for extra medication if your pain has increased.

One important tip: Because constipation is inevitable when taking any narcotic, implement a plan for relieving constipation from the beginning. In addition to a stool softener, laxative, or other recommendation, include good portions of vegetables, fruit, and salad in your daily meals, above and beyond the tablets you will be given. If the fruits and vegetables on your hospital tray look unappetizing, ask family or friends to bring you fresh fruit and veggies from home.

Coughing and Deep-Breathing Exercises

Your healthcare team will be teaching you breathing exercises and coughing techniques. Yes, both of these will hurt at first. In many hospitals a special pillow—in my case, a large, red, heart-shaped pillow—will be offered to hug to your chest in order to support the sore incision. This helps! Do everything you can to get into the swing of taking deep breaths through a small plastic device, so your team can monitor the increasing force of your breath, then coughing as strongly as possible to keep your lungs clear.

Walking with Support Stockings

Walking—at intervals per your doctor's instructions—is very good for you. As your strength increases, you will be urged to walk longer and farther along the hospital's corridors. You will need to wear tightly woven, elastic, knee-length support stockings. They support the legs without interfering with circulation, and they help prevent fluid from accumulating in the legs and causing them to swell. Check with your doctor to see how many more weeks the support hose should be worn, at least during the day, once you are home.

Eating Well and Keeping Up Your Appetite

The first meal presented to you at the hospital will probably not make you salivate. So often hospital food continues to live up to its poor reputation. Add to that the heart-healthy aspect of meals served on any cardiac wing (with low or no sodium), and you may be facing a series of dull, unappetizing meals. That said, it is nevertheless very important to take in good quantities of nourishing food and liquids to speed the healing of your incision and your traumatized body as a whole. Your surgeon has probably ordered a standard diet, but modifications can be made in consultation with the hospital's dietician, who may also offer a diet class at the hospital that you and your caregiver can attend. In addition, you might ask a family member to pick up healthy beverage and food treats to augment the hospital menu.

Personalizing Your Temporary Environment

While spending your week or so in the hospital, consider livening up your surroundings. Here's what caregiver Beth did to desterilize and cheer up her husband's temporary quarters:

I took photographs I already had of our life together and the people most important to us (grandchild, friends, and such) and blew them up on a color copier and hung them on the hospital room's wall for him to look at and feel encouraged to come back to himself. The side benefit of putting up all these color photos was that then the staff began to know something about who we were, as individuals and as a couple. I think the photographs made a huge difference in the level of care my husband received from nurses, lab techs, and other personnel.

Being Wise about Visitors

Both in the hospital and later at home, visits from friends and family can be buoying and energizing, but they can also be exhausting. People should be asked to check in before coming to see you, and both you and your caregiver should be prepared to decline, or to pace and suggest time limits for these visits.

Countering Anxiety and the Blues

Periods of feeling anxious or "blue" are part of the process of recovery. Even as we are working hard at our routine of week-after-surgery assignments—walking, resting, coughing, deep breathing, attending patient education classes—we are superalert to our emotions and the constant chatter in our heads. We worry that any new physical twinge may be a setback, and simply because we have been through so much already, a feeling of depression can be temporarily triggered by relatively small things. I was lucky to have family members giving me a lot of love and support in the hospital, but I still spent a bad evening of distress and anxiety trying to get the attention of a night nurse who was too occupied with an urgent situation to answer my call.

In the short term, the best antidote to counter these emotions is communication. As feelings of anxiety arise, talk about them with a caring nurse or family members. Remember that this is an emotionally trying time for your caregiver too, so allow yourselves to loosen your everyday emotional controls and share your feelings with each other.

Bottom line: it's important to know that periods of depression can arise at any time and in most cases remain only temporarily. In the moment, don't hesitate to consult your doctor, physician's assistant, or another member of the hospital team for help in managing your feelings, including, perhaps, taking short-term antidepressant medication. (For information on dealing with less transient symptoms of depression, see "Keep an Eye Out for Symptoms of Depression" on pages 94–95 and "Emotional Ups and Downs" on pages 155–158.)

Reclaiming Your Vulnerable Independence

Recovery from an open-heart operation, if it's to be swift and optimal, demands that the patient take a stand for personal self-care and independence. Even a gifted cardiologist can do just so much for you. It's patients who take an active role—by being honest with themselves about how they feel, acting on their feelings by asking questions and getting help, committing to stick to healthier lifestyle choices (which is difficult to do)— who create the optimal conditions for successful recoveries.

Taking this kind of responsibility for oneself means agreeing to work with personal discomfort, both physical and mental. Not everyone is up for this. For every patient who relishes taking control, who follows a self-made walking-resting-breathing schedule and reports any concerns to their medical team, there is another patient for whom reestablishing self-reliance is a challenge. Ultimately, your returning health depends upon your attitude. Just as it takes about one month to deliberately break a habit if we commit to positive thinking and action on a daily basis, we can also retrain our thinking to welcome the gift of returning heart health, discomforts and all. Though still feeling vulnerable, work in partnership with everyone on your medical team. Defer to doctors' instructions but always be ready to ask questions about what concerns you. In other words, even while you're still in the hospital, be cooperative yet vigilant.

The Flurry of Discharge Instructions

Suddenly, when you are about to be discharged, a flurry of activity occurs, including visits from hospital staff you haven't seen in a while and even some you have never met before. An exercise physiologist may come to demonstrate prescribed daily workouts. A dietician may swoop in to review dietary requirements. You can probably expect one last check-in by your surgeon and any attending physicians. Your day nurse or the physician's assistant will give you a rundown on the detailed home instruction packet.

Do your best to take it all in. Save any materials you are given. And if you have particular concerns because of a complication that arose in the hospital or something else that worries you, make sure you and your caregiver inquire about *exactly* what to expect at home. A home care advisory nurse may be available for this important discussion. Try to leave with every one of your questions answered, but don't hesitate to call upon anyone on the hospital team for consultations or links to other appropriate healthcare professionals who can give you support after you've returned home.

Reducing Stress on the Caregiver

Once the hospital is in the rearview mirror, suddenly being in charge of everything can be overwhelming for the primary caregiver. This person has already put in days of sharing the patient's worries along with giving major practical support, including overtime doing household chores, additional research, note-taking, and scheduling to keep the recovery process moving forward. Caregivers often arrive at the hospital discharge moment quite exhausted. They carry a tremendous burden, yet for the most part the system is not designed to take them into account.

So getting practical, compassionate support going into the home recovery phase is vital for the caregiver as well, which is why a home team can be so sustaining. As many caregivers have made clear to me, stress is inherent in the role of supporter.

Here are a few hospital discharge suggestions from Sherry, who was her husband Jim's primary caregiver when he had a mitral valve repair at age seventy-two:

- Ask the hospital pharmacist to give you both the generic and the original brand names of all medications the patient will be taking during recovery. In the event of arthritic hands, or out of sheer preference, ask for non-childproof caps.
- Invite a second person to accompany you when the patient is released from the hospital, especially if you will be loaded down with more than your overnight bags—like an oxygen canister, a box containing a raised toilet seat, or other special equipment.
- Arrange to have a meal or snack ready for you as soon as you arrive home.

A few weeks later, Sherry had these final words of advice:

Call on your reserves of patience. Be prepared for mood swings! If the patient has never been dependent before, be prepared to be resented. Jim had his outbursts! One time, for example, I didn't unlock the car door fast enough as he was trying to get in. There are trying moments...

Information You Need Before Checking Out

- Who can you call 24/7 and under what circumstances should you call 911? Leave the hospital with specific guidelines about emergencies and a list of names and phone numbers to access when you have less urgent concerns, including contacts who can be called at night or on weekends.

- Together with your caregiver, be clear which medications to take *when* and *for how long*.

- Know when to schedule your first post-op appointment with either your surgeon or a local doctor.

- Ask about the *psychological* challenges you will face, above and beyond the physical take-home instructions (incision care, medical equipment, pain management, diet, activities, and so forth).

- Ask for specific tips for countering caregiver stress.

- Finally, is there one last question that's just occurred to you? If so, ask it before you leave.

Part Three

Managing Your Recovery
at Home

CHAPTER EIGHT

Losing and Regaining Spiritual Strength

A Personal Perspective

I'VE COME TO BELIEVE THAT, metaphorically speaking, there were angels surrounding my open-heart surgery experience. Much as I fought the impending event, I sensed I was never alone. In the months leading up to the operation, whenever I was able to pause, meditate, and relax into a quiet, peaceful state of mind, a caring presence seemed always nearby. And although I hadn't always been aware of it during my childhood or while I was immersed in raising a family, coping with divorce, and establishing a career, I now know that this caring presence has always been there for me.

Losing and regaining spiritual strength is a thread that has woven through my life at various intensities as far back as I can remember. Recently at an Adult Congenital Heart Association conference (ACHA), cardiologist William Davidson, director of the adult congenital heart disease division at Penn State's Medical Center, told me that Ebstein's Anomaly was "an odd duck, an anomaly all by itself" amidst the array of the thirty-five known congenital heart defects. Did this explain, I wondered, why as a child I had often felt like an utterly unique specimen of a human, different from everyone else? Maybe we all feel this way, at least to some degree. But in retrospect I had a tangible reason to feel I was different: I had a structural heart defect.

Here's what it was like growing up with a sense that there was something peculiar about me that separated me from others. Before I was even in school I remember my parents taking me to the dimly lit New York City office of creaky Dr. Schloss for an electrocardiogram. Dr. Schloss whispered. In fact, everyone in the office whispered. My worried parents, following suit, were barely audible to me. And, with so little light or sound in that office, how could I interpret their obvious anxiety?

I felt further disconnected from others and my own sense of well-being at age five, upon learning that Dr. Schloss had died. His death upset me profoundly. Death was an eerie concept at such a young age. By association, could I be next?

Every year after that, my mother took me to the Yale-New Haven Medical Center in New Haven, Connecticut, to see Dr. Ruth Whitamore, a pediatric cardiology special-ist. And once, when my mother and I sat in the waiting room for our appointment, an odd-looking child—his eyes not in the right places—sat down across from us with his mother. I was frightened. Was there something *that* wrong with me too? Today I know that the child must have had Down's syndrome, which is often accompanied by one or more congenital heart defects. But how was I to put this all together at the age of nine?

My spiritual moorings were challenged more deeply as a teenager, when Dr. Whitamore warned me that I might not be able to have children; pregnancy, she explained, could overstress my structurally challenged heart. She wasn't posi-tive, however. We'd wait and see. Having already internalized the belief that I might not make it to adulthood, I was dev-astated. Then the late 1950s ushered in cardiac catheteriza-tion, which enabled precise measurements to be taken of the severity of my condition, revealing that my heart functions were only "mildly" disturbed. As long as I agreed to be fol-lowed by a cardiologist, I was assured, pregnancy would be viable for me. To my great joy, my early worries had been put to rest and my life felt spirituallly blessed. Not only could I anticipate a vital adulthood, but now it might include the prospect of children.

A new sense of spiritual awakening occurred again a few years before the progression of my Ebstein's made it neces-sary to consider open-heart surgery. Then, having made the decision, I followed a program of preparation that had a spiritual component at its base. I put in hours using Peggy Huddleston's *Prepare for Surgery, Heal Faster* relaxation tape, and I composed affirmations envisioning positive outcomes for my surgery. A loving group of spiritual practitioner friends, along with the minister of our church, offered me a prayer session by phone a few days before my surgery date. Other friends were lined up for dinner deliveries once I returned home. And before the operation I was regularly in touch with a terrific online support group. All this advance preparation had strengthened my spirit and my sense of oneness with everyone. Then, unexpectedly, during the first week I was home I became overwhelmed. Significant emotional and physical challenges presented themselves, and my high spirits caved.

My spiritual vigor—rooted in my deep-seated sense that God is all there is and that I am an individualized expression of the infinity of God, restrained only by my own limiting beliefs—collapsed, went underground, was lost to me. Where had my sense of connectedness gone now that I was home?

Though I didn't realize it at the time, it began to escape me ever so slightly during my postsurgery week in the hospital. Because I had taken such good care to prepare myself for the frightening surgery, and experienced such relief once out the other side, my family and I were elated. Every time my surgeon and his entourage swept through I wanted them to know how remarkably well I was doing. I wanted to stand out as a larger-than-life example, the exceptional heart surgery patient. In other words, my ego claimed the day.

A week later I traveled by plane from Rochester to Minneapolis, Minneapolis south to Albuquerque, and then seventy more miles by car to Santa Fe. Nothing had seemed odd about that. My surgeon and everyone else thought I would be fine, based on how enthusiastically I was relating to them. I was wheel-chaired through security to the airplane's open door to preserve my fragile energy, but actually I wanted to jump out and sing!—or at least walk on my own through the airport.

It was this exuberance that fooled me into overdoing everything once I was back home. Without checking in with myself to assess how I *really* felt, I willed my way through phone conversations that lasted way too long, or through the assigned shoulder flexion and rotation exercises no matter how tired I was. I sat in the back seat of the car, not in the front passenger seat (too close to an airbag), complaining to my husband about the car-riding restriction (at that time) as he drove me to my first post-op appointment. The nurse in charge, astonished that I was up and about just ten days after my surgery, made a statement I will never forget: "Above all, don't let yourself get discouraged. I hear that's really the challenge for open-heart surgery recovery."

Me, get discouraged? I thought. No way.

Because I was wrapped up in my own self-care (and a certain amount of pouting), it was only later that I realized what had been going on—that, without meaning to,

I had turned my back on the spiritual practices that had so nourished me. As a result, I had been taking the generically written hospital discharge instructions literally: look after the incision; avoid pushing, pulling, or lifting more than five or ten pounds; avoid fatigue by balancing rest with activities; and so on. I paid attention to little else. Each instruction in the discharge materials I had gotten was typically composed of one sentence, with no embellishment, no human touch. The prize phrase was "expect both good and bad days." Here, I later told myself, is where a juicy paragraph should have been included! What is home recovery *really* like? *Mention* how blue a recovering patient can feel, that there is the possibility of temporary depression; *mention* that there may be memory challenges (usually short–term ones); *mention* that the fatigue can be more intense and drawn out than any fatigue you have ever experienced before. Warn us, in these instructions, that open-heart surgery recovery has unique psychological challenges as well as physical ones!

In the first weeks after my return home, I did not get back to my morning routine of reading daily guides and affirmations. I had shut the door on this enjoyable and sustaining spiritual activity. I did write in my personal journal, but without regularity. I didn't go online to connect with my support group. Nor did I pursue any of the open-heart surgery recovery tips I'd read about in books. Although Bill was extremely attentive and caring, I didn't invite camaraderie or support from friends, even when they stopped by to leave us dinner. Weakened by my as yet undiagnosed anemia, I could handle visits from outsiders for no longer than five or ten minutes at a time. Where now was that benign presence, that sense of connection, when all I felt was lousy?

What had been showing up was depression—something that never occurred to me. I was simply too positive a person, and too proud of my positive attitude, to consider that depression could invade my psychic space. But of course, our physical and psychological health are intertwined, which is why it's important to tune in to what both body and psyche are telling us.

There was a period, about three weeks after returning home, when it was clear I was going downhill, not up. My primary care physician was out of town, and the doctor I met with was feeling ill herself. She almost rescheduled the appointment, but thought better of disappointing me. Although she asked some good questions when we met, her knowledge about post-op issues for open-heart surgery patients was limited. And while sympathetic regarding my intense fatigue and more recent low-grade fever, she didn't think to run blood tests to see if I might be anemic. (Anemia, it turns out, is common after heart surgery.) She did ask, however, if I would like to take home samples of an antidepression medication. I, of course (in my know-it-all state), turned that down.

Meanwhile, I dragged myself around the house, angry and frustrated, wondering if I would ever return to my old self. As luck would have it—indeed, I count it as a touch of grace—I spoke on the phone with someone who had been sent home from open-heart surgery with iron tablets as a matter of course. I called my physician's office and insisted on a blood count and other tests to get to the bottom of my fever and exhaustion. A visit with my cardiologist one month past surgery revealed the reason for my low-grade fever (pericarditis, an inflammation of the sac that encloses the heart). And the blood count confirmed that I was anemic. It took two weeks for them to kick in, but the iron tablets brought my blood count—and my energy level—back into the normal range.

At about the four-and-a-half-week point, once my body temperature had returned to normal and iron was replenishing my strength, strands of mental clarity began beaming their way through. My inner spiritual connection, the caring presence I'd sensed before, was in evidence again as well. Suddenly, at five weeks, I was brimming with ideas for a "wish-I-knew-beforehand" list and a new sense of purpose. I was writing in my journal regularly, with the idea of documenting my progress in order to share advice with other heart patients. I was consciously, deliberately, into surrender—to "letting go and letting God." Finally I was hearing what my more spiritual friends had been reminding me: sometimes we have a certain amount of control over our circumstances and sometimes we simply do not.

I wish I had known, during that first recovery month, how to keep my spiritual connection alive. But in reality, it is so daunting to be home, on your own, facing physical and emotional challenges, that one can easily feel overwhelmed and forget to ask for help.

So, okay. Forgive yourself. Now—whenever "now" appears —pick up the phone and reach out for what you need.

CHAPTER NINE

Home Sweet Home— Maybe

 HALLELUJAH, YOU'RE HOME! You have made remarkable progress since the surgery, otherwise you wouldn't be here.

But wait. You're weary. And so is your caregiver.

A Reminder for Caregivers

You've been living on adrenalin for days now, and a sense of overwhelm is creeping in. All that ready-made medical advice you were getting in the hospital is no longer at your fingertips. Yes, you have phone numbers to call. But there are so *many* items in the take-home instructions for you to supervise—how will you manage it all? Help! I have a baby elephant on my hands!

It's normal to feel flustered and on edge once you realize just how huge a responsibility you're facing. Consider lining up help and support if you haven't already. No apologies necessary. The first two to four weeks are especially trying times for the caregiver as well as the patient. Because the fatigue of first-phase recovery is so intense—a patient tires quickly, frequently needs to rest, and gets discouraged—you may soon become run-down yourself if you don't ask for help.

You might find you've participated in the phenomenon of thinking, If I can *just get through* the surgery with my loved one, I'll be home free. Similarly, the patient has been thinking, If I can *just get through* the operation and wake up alive, the rest is a piece of cake. Not so. The hard work of recovery lies ahead. A professional colleague of mine who emigrated to the United States from Romania draws a parallel: she describes how immigrants who have grown up under Communism kiss the ground when they arrive in America, then get sideswiped by the hardships they encounter in assimilating into the new culture. If you haven't done so already, it's time to acknowledge that there is a long, winding road ahead for both you and your convalescing patient. Plan to treat yourself to caring support from others. (See Chapter 4 for specific suggestions.)

Here is an encouraging comment from Beth, a caregiver quoted in previous chapters:

> I turned to three close and dear friends who were on call for me for weeks and weeks. Even though two of them are geographically so far away that they couldn't offer physical help, their quality of listening made a huge difference for me.

The Importance of Pacing

For the patient, learning to adjust to what you can handle without pushing yourself so hard that you risk a major setback, is the secret to a good recovery from open-heart surgery. Remember that each person's recovery is different. How active you were before surgery and the nature of the operation you have had are two factors that will affect your recovery time.

It will be six to eight weeks before many of the post-op instructions you were given will no longer need your attention. As much as six months later your body still will not have entirely forgotten its ordeal. No matter how well your surgery has gone, you have been through a formidable experience. It takes time, patience, and a positive attitude to get to the point where you can pick up your life again from where you left off. The secret lies in pacing yourself wisely.

Typical Instructions and Common Problems

While it can be extremely helpful to compare notes with other recovering open-heart patients—by phone for instance, or in a support group—remember that no two recoveries will look the same. Instructions for resuming challenging activities (using the treadmill, driving, lifting a thirty-pound toddler) are unique for each of us. The following, in alphabetical order, is a "watch list" of some of the items you will be monitoring, with cross-references to additional discussions in this book. Where cross-references are not given, please refer to the publications, associations, or online resources listed at the back of the book.

First and foremost, follow your doctor's written and verbal directions regarding all activities. And *take the initiative* to ask questions of your designated medical liaison at any time.

- **Anger and depression:** Many patients are unprepared for bouts of irritability, unexplainable sadness, chronic tiredness, sleeping difficulties, sudden weeping, and so on—all normal reactions to the trauma of major surgery that should be transient and gradually disappear within about three months. If they are either troublesome or persistent, see your doctor and consider seeking counseling. (For more about what to watch for, see "Keep an Eye Out for Symptoms of Depression" on pages 94–95 and "Emotional Ups and Downs" on pages 155–158.)

- **Appetite:** Your appetite may take a dive, but it will pick up. (See "Eating Well and Keeping Up Your Appetite" on page 113 for short-term advice). When it does, treat yourself to a heart-healthy cookbook and look for recipes that involve making minimal changes to *what* you like to eat, but offer healthier ways to prepare particular meals.

- **Being active:** It takes time to get your strength back after surgery. You'll want to walk every day, per your doctor's instructions—aiming to increase the time by five minutes a day, for example. But if this doesn't suit you yet, take it easier. There are many low-stress activities you can enjoy around the house, including meal planning and preparation, board or card games, potting plants, minor home repairs, needle-work, reading, and personal hobbies. Get dressed every day, stay involved with life, and be as active as you can.

- **Cardiac rehabilitation programs:** Having had an excellent experience at my local cardiac rehabilitation facility, I am a big fan of joining a program after several weeks have passed. These programs provide camaraderie and teach recovering heart patients how to exercise safely, while monitoring you closely so that you won't run into trouble. (See "Beginning a Cardiac Rehab Program—Eureka!" on pages 158–160.)

- **Driving:** Honor your doctor's instructions not to drive for four to six weeks. Your breastbone, now held together by wire sutures, is still extremely vulnerable, and even a very small accident with you in the driver's seat could slam your chest into the steering wheel. (See "Driving and Lifting Restrictions" on pages 98–99 for information about being a passenger.)

- **Incisions:** Much of your initial discomfort may be in the area of your incisions. You might feel sore (or numb, or itchy) along the line that runs up and down the center of your chest, or soreness along a leg or abdomen incision. Follow your surgeon's or nurse's instructions on how to care for your incisions, so they will remain free of infection and heal quickly. Call your medical liaison person with any questions or concerns.

- **Insomnia:** Sleeplessness can occur for many reasons, especially when you can't get physically comfortable. If you have problems getting enough rest, contact your medical liaison person for advice and perhaps a prescription for a sleep aid.

- **Medications:** You may be sent home with only one prescription for pain relief, or with many for various purposes. It's important to know which medications you should take and how often. See "The Medication Potpourri" on pages 146–147 for important guidelines about side effects and managing a mix. (See also "Discuss the Issue of Pain Management" on pages 76–77, "Allergic Reactions, Pain Medication Side Effects, and Drug Interactions" on page 91, and "Accepting Pain Relief" on pages 111–112.)

- **Memory loss:** Memory loss and general mental fuzziness are usually temporary. (See "Cognitive Issues" on page 96 and "Lingering Cognitive Challenges" on pages 149–151 for more information.)

- **Pushing, pulling, lifting:** Moving your arms in the simplest way will let you know immediately that your chest muscles are *very* tender! Above all, you will have been directed not to put any kind of even indirect strain on your healing breastbone for six weeks. This means steering clear of trying to open stuck windows, unscrew jammed jar lids, and lift grocery bags, children, pets, or suitcases. (See Chapter 4 for tips on how to deal with this temporary disability.)

- **Relaxation and coping techniques:** Coping techniques that are easy to experiment with in the early days of recovery, especially when feeling blue, are listed on pages 157–158. Additional avenues to explore include acupuncture, Reiki, massage, stretching and deep-breathing exercises, writing or journaling, drawing or painting.

- **Rest:** Routines like showering, towel-drying yourself, and brushing your hair will be quite tiring at first. Your body responds to all activities now as "work." Give in and rest at least twice a day, not necessarily sleeping, or even in bed, but with your feet up. (See "The Impatient Patient" on pages 151–155.)

- **Sex:** What *will* become of our sex lives, most of us want to know. It's a topic often treated humorously, as in the 2003 Diane Keaton and Jack Nicholson movie *Something's Got to Give*. Nicholson's "movie" doctor said, if after his heart attack he could climb two flights of stairs, he was ready for sex. It was hilarious to watch him repeatedly test himself. Seriously, don't hesitate to contact your doctor with your questions and concerns about resuming sexual activity. As with everything else, you will be encouraged to begin gradually and to communicate fears and discomforts candidly with your partner. So relax and laugh together and keep in close touch.

- **Support stockings:** Support stockings may strike you as a nuisance when you are introduced to them in the hospital, but they are a reinforcing invention. They facilitate blood flow, particularly in the beginning weeks of your recovery, before you are walking regularly and activating your leg muscles.

• **Visitors:** Visitors mean well, but their attention can exhaust you. Here is where pacing your daily routine, one day at a time, including limiting the time you spend on phone calls and answering email, can make all the difference. (See "Designate a Follow-up Communicator" on pages 85–86 and "Being Wise about Visitors" on page 114.)

• **When to call the doctor:** Happily, far fewer serious post-operative complications pop up than ever before. While it's important to use common sense, heart patients and caregivers should not hesitate to seek medical advice when questions arise. Even when it comes to interpreting your take-home instructions involving a simple answer, if you're uncertain, pick up the phone and get clarification.

• **When to call 911:** You will be given a list of serious symptoms to watch out for during your home recovery, which you should review regularly, yet the unexpected may also occur. Any time you think you are experiencing a sudden, seemingly severe medical challenge, call 911. (My own postsurgery ER experience involving emergency symptoms appears in "The Impatient Patient" on pages 151–155.)

• **Work:** You will undoubtedly have had several conversations with your medical team about when to suspend and resume work. Now that you're in the recovery period, you'll need to pay attention to your own body in order to know when you are ready for work or not, depending in part on your job's requirements (sedentary as opposed to more physically taxing). In any case, best to resume working little by little, part-time at first, and to keep alert for overdoing it as you test your thresholds. As a life coaching principle encourages, you'll want to be able to underpromise yourself and overdeliver.

CHAPTER TEN

More on the Jagged Progress Forward

"YOU CAN EXPECT BOTH GOOD DAYS and bad days," Mayo Clinic personnel cheerfully inform post–open-heart surgery patients. The take-home patient education manual offers the same advice. I'm all for taking an upbeat approach, but for many of us this is a serious understatement. From my own experience and that of numerous heart patients I've talked to, the first two or three weeks at home can be so trying that a patient may doubt whether the operation was worth it. Fortunately, periods of mental fogginess, temporary memory loss, and intense fatigue, plus challenges with pain meds and generally drooping spirits, are punctuated with hours of grateful positive feelings and a sense of slowly returning to "humanhood." It's important to remember, though, that the progress forward is jagged, not linear.

Recuperation Is Your Full-Time Job

So now you are home, and while the healing process is well underway—or you would not have been discharged from the hospital—there are miles to go. There seem to be so many instructions to remember. You simply will not be up to much in the first few weeks, and in some cases you won't be able to do a lot of what you're used to being able to do for several more. Yes, an upbeat approach by the hospital medical staff may have sent you waltzing home, but while it's thrilling to be leaving the hospital, where you haven't been permitted to sleep through the night, still you are returning home greatly fatigued, with a medications schedule to manage, possibly a tank of oxygen, and perhaps recurrent irregular heartbeats or other complications that remain unresolved. Now is the time to dedicate yourself to the hard work of recovery. Alternating rest and exercise, and above all, *patience* with the physical and emotional trials ahead, is your assignment for the next several weeks.

Combining Preparation, Vigilance, and Patience

You and your caregiver will mostly be on your own unless your particular situation requires a treatment plan that includes post-op visits from a home healthcare nurse. Even if that's the case, now is the time to reread Chapter 5, "The Challenges You May Face," and to review any guidelines your hospital medical team has given you about things to watch out for. Whenever in doubt about what you may be experiencing, contact your designated medical liaison for professional diagnosis or medical attention. *No question or concern is too trivial.*

Every recovery is different. If you've been told to expect improvement "two days forward, one day back," you might be disappointed to experience instead only one good day (a period of energetic spunk) followed by two, three, or even four days of just plain feeling lousy. Even to meet the assignment of increasing your walking time from five minutes to ten minutes a day may feel like an insurmountable task at first. You may be swinging in and out of depression. (See Chapter 5, and "Emotional Ups and Downs" on pages 155–158.) You may feel "off" and think you are coming down with a virus, and while that might be the case, feeling off can be due to other things as well: you may have become anemic (as I did), or succumbed to an allergic reaction, or sleep deprivation may have caught up with you. Know that everyone goes through discouragement, yet those who *expect* the ups and downs will fare better. Trust that in several weeks your strength will turn a major corner, and so for the short term if you are worried, contact the appropriate member of your follow-up care team.

With regard to the issue of patience, I discovered a trick for getting through these weeks: invite an affirmative mental attitude to accompany you. Take stock daily—maybe by gazing out your window in simple contemplation—and remind yourself of all the good in your life, of everyone and everything you are grateful for. Try to continuously refresh the notion that you are in a *temporary* state of mind and body. You *are* healing, and yes, the process may seem slow, redundant, but you will come to a point—or several points—where you will notice significant stamina has returned.

Such an exercise in patience is something not all of us are good at. (It was certainly a challenge for me.) To get better at it, affirm small positive recovery results every day and reach out for appealing and comforting activities: cook up tempting (and healthy) meals, choose locations to do your walking in fresh air, plan low-key outings (with your next nap at home in mind), indulge yourself with inspirational music and books, a game of Scrabble, comedy movie rentals, giggly conversations with your nearest and dearest. You will definitely experience cabin fever during this long recovery period, so please give yourself permission to spoil yourself silly. Indulge in a weekly massage at home, rent a comfy recliner, hire a musician to serenade you and your caregiver for dinner, plan your next vacation and begin the reservation process.

The Medication Potpourri

While some heart surgery patients are sent home with just pain relievers and aspirin, others face the challenge of managing a potpourri of prescriptions. We live in a world of advanced wonder drugs—that's the good news. But our bodies produce unique physical responses, particularly to combinations of prescription and over-the-counter meds together with supplements. Some potential interactions between medications are well-known and clinically documented, whereas others are not. And your own particular body has experience with some medication combinations and not others. So there is a chance you will respond negatively to anything new in the mix. Consult with your healthcare professional about side effects and drug interactions and whether a particular response might be a sign of sensitivity, an inflammation, or an allergic reaction. In *The Cardiac Recovery Handbook*, Dr. Paul Kligfield advises the following:

> It can be very confusing to keep track of the cocktail of medications that your doctor has probably prescribed for you. Before you go home, make sure you know:
> - The names of your medications (it may be helpful to note both generic and brand name to avoid confusion when you go to the pharmacy)
> - What it does
> - How much to take
> - When and how to take it
> - What the possible side effects of each medication are
> - What to do if you forget and miss a pill

Sample Days

During the first week home, you won't believe how long it takes to do everything. Say you wake up at 7:30 a.m. Gingerly you position your elbows to haul yourself out of bed. Before going into the bathroom it's a good idea to alert your caregiver that you're up, especially if you're planning to take a shower. (If your caregiver sleeps in a different part of the house, you might consider using walkie-talkies.) By the time you're dressed, you're ready to lie down again to rest! The following day you might opt for breakfast before showering, shaving, or putting on makeup. However you slice it, first thing in the morning you'll need to ask for help putting on the elastic support stockings you'll be wearing daily for the next three weeks. It's very hard on your tender chest muscles to tug them on yourself.

To visualize each day with positive purpose, begin the morning by checking the medication and exercise chart you will have made for yourself. From breakfast to lunch, you'll be alternating rest and activity. You may be drawn to the morning paper, a TV show, or your computer. Inevitably you will do too much until learning to anticipate the need for rest *before* you're wiped out. Because you want to feel normal, you may dally at the computer too long, as I did. Returning to bed or sofa for a mere fifteen minutes of quiet, with feet up, will give you renewed energy. The next time up, run through some simple upper-body arm movements—the physical therapy routine you designed with the help of your nurse or the PA before leaving the hospital. Include your breathing exercises, then settle down again, before fatigue recurs, to relax with that special book or some music, TV, or radio. Before lunch, walk around the house for five minutes on the exercise circuit you've mapped out for yourself.

For a week or two, your afternoons will be similar to your mornings. You'll plan to rest regularly, perhaps even doze (although you don't want to overdo napping, particularly later in the afternoon, because it may hinder a good night's sleep) and chat regularly on the phone with good friends. You might also want to get peer support from a former or currently recovering heart patient—to compare notes, become allies. Being with friends is a good thing, but invite them for brief fifteen-to-thirty-minute visits only; even happy, spirited conversing can be exhausting. Walk another five-minute round. Rest again. Repeat the breathing exercises again. Anticipate dinner with relish. In the evening, check your medication-activities chart, honor your accomplishments for the day, and plan for the next. At bedtime, after the video or the music or the book or the TV show, you will need to ask your partner or caregiver to remove the support hose for you.

With not much changing day after day at first, you'll want to be as creative as you can with all that homebound rest time. Keep a journal or a progress diary. Give yourself over to projects that you've spent months wishing you'd had the time for. Create that photo album, enjoy crossword puzzles. Experiment with a new hobby. Gently reemerge yourself in a fraction of your work. If the weather cooperates, begin to take your short walks outside; otherwise, walk in a mall. As time goes on and your tolerance for activity increases, your need for frequent resting periods will decrease.

Lingering Cognitive Challenges
While making great efforts to complete your physical assignments every day—to balance walking, resting, napping,

stretching, eating, and socializing—you may well be grap-
pling with mental irritants as well. In an article in the October 4, 2004 issue of the *Los Angeles Times*, titled "Heal the
Heart, Hurt the Mind?" Judy Foreman writes that, possibly
due to being hooked up to a heart-lung machine, some open-
heart surgery patients "find that their brains don't function as
well as they did before. These effects can dissipate in a few
days or continue for months or [more likely in older patients]
for years."

The culprit? Although it is suspected, Foreman continues,
it is *not* clear that the cause is the patient's time spent on the
heart-lung machine. The "pump head" theory she's referring
to postulates that "when the heart is stopped during surgery…
small blood clots, air bubbles and other debris" are "traveling
to the brain and disrupting memory." In recent years, some
cardiac surgeons have become advocates for "off-pump" heart
surgery, which is now used in 22 percent of coronary bypass
procedures. Foreman quotes Dr. John Puskas, an associate pro-
fessor in the division of cardiothoracic surgery at Emory University in Atlanta, as saying, "I think it's clear that off-pump
is better, but proving it with scientific rigor is challenging"; a
study from Johns Hopkins that Foreman also cites found no
difference in patients' cognitive outcomes that could be attributed to whether they'd had their surgery on- or off-pump. The
point is, for each of us, that open-heart surgery recovery is
going to have its grueling moments. And through the early
weeks at home, a great portion of the challenge may be mental
or psychological, not just physical.

Another perspective is expressed by Denys Cope, RN, BSN, a healthcare case manager in Santa Fe, New Mexico. She suggests that it can take a full six months for general anesthesia to completely leave the body and thus it is the lingering anesthesia that can temporarily impair cognitive function. Detoxing from anesthesia, she adds, can often be accelerated with acupuncture or a homeopathic remedy.

My personal theory? How about the sheer stress of just plain undergoing open-heart surgery? The assault to the physical body alone for me felt larger than any imaginable physical disorientation. I attributed my mental fogginess to oppressive fatigue—a unique trademark of heart surgery that is unlike any other fatigue. In addition, I became anemic three weeks after surgery and dragged around for another two weeks until the iron pills kicked in. This development, plus surgical intrusion into my heart weeks before, surely impacted my brain. Although we can't capture and label it for certain, expect a distinctive brand of "la-la land" effect meandering through your physical activities for several days or weeks. And keep reminding yourself: this too shall pass!

The Impatient Patient
The most difficult lesson for me during my healing was to learn to listen to my body and not ignore a message I didn't like. For example, in the beginning of my recovery it was clear I needed to lie down or nap frequently. Two or three weeks into recovery, I thought I should feel improved. *Should* is the culprit here. My surgeon and his assistant had

both said to expect a slow recovery, to accept the "two days forward, one day back" cycle. So what about the *two* days backward, even three or four? What about picking up a bug because the immune system is so compromised? As it turns out, the more rest we consciously pursue during open-heart surgery recovery, the smoother the healing process will be.

I remember our housekeeper, who had undergone surgery the year before, kept harping at me to rest, rest, rest. I would say, Yes, I know, I know. But did I rest as much as I might have? I see now that I could have taken it a *lot* easier: less playing at my computer, and more time lying on the bed or couch reading. A dear friend who'd had major surgery had told me she'd broken all records and healed completely in three weeks, not the six predicted. I would do that too! I had secretly declared to myself. I was completely healthy going into my tricuspid valve repair surgery, I was not "sick." I intended to heal in three weeks also. If she could do it, I could do it.

Well, she and I are different physical beings. Nor was hers open-heart surgery, which is known to have a lengthier recuperation period than other procedures. I knew that, but it was not easy for me to *give in,* to rest, impromptu, when the body called, even though every time I did so I felt restored.

There was a more serious side to this tug-of-war around honoring my body, however. The struggle showed up as wanting to let go—agreeing to surrender to my healing path's natural pacing—versus my habitual drive to *will* something into being, to *will* myself better. So about a month after my surgery I composed a convincing journal entry on letting my process just be. "I allow God to be the cocreator of my healing with me," I wrote. "My recovery will progress exactly the way it is meant to go. I will listen to—and respect—my body's wishes and needs. I will keep checking that still, small voice inside…"

However, the following day I wound up in the emergency room. Instead of reminding myself of what my physicians told me—that it would take up to three months before I would no longer go into atrial fibrillation (the irregular heart rhythm) from time to time—I had decided to take matters into my own hands. I was five weeks past surgery. I was experiencing this annoying heart rhythm pretty regularly. That day, when the atrial fibrillation returned, I made a judgment that was really an irresponsible guess: I reasoned that since taking a big dose of the anti-arrhythmic medication, followed by a second big dose an hour later, had worked well to arrest my a-fib *before* having surgery, I could try this route again. *I'll* take control! I thought. *I* will revert my a-fib back to normal heart rhythm.

Instead, I overdosed. An hour or two later my heartbeat dropped to a dangerously low level. Feeling lousy, I recorded a heart rhythm reading on my portable "event monitor" device. Then, as before, I dialed the 800 number, placed the telephone mouthpiece on the monitor's speaker, and transmitted the recording over the phone line to the supervising lab. The cardiologist on call that weekend phoned back immediately. "Your very low heart rate concerns me, and I can't assess what's going on over the phone. I strongly recommend you come into the ER to be evaluated." The recording I'd transmitted had signaled heart block—a condition that slows down, or blocks, the electrical impulses that need to travel freely through the heart.

Minutes later, I could not sit up in bed. I had no strength to even move. Lying there I realized I couldn't make it to the car, and I asked Bill to call 911. I felt the energy draining out of me fast, as if I were dying...

The local fire-and-rescue team arrived in no time with three vehicles, including an ambulance. (I was lucky, because the volunteers were running a practice session nearby.) It seemed like ten guys showed up in our bedroom! They trailed in all their heart-monitoring equipment, beepers, cell phones, oxygen, stretcher—et al. The huge amount of energy emanating from them was almost unbearable for me to handle, yet we made it to the hospital and got my heart block episode taken care of in the nick of time.

I learned an important lesson that day: There is a lot I can control and a lot I cannot possibly control. We know what we know, and we know some of what we don't know. I am not a physician. Medical divination is not one of my talents. The big dose of anti-arrhythmic medication after the onset of atrial fibrillation, had been prescribed a year earlier by my original electrophysiologist; had I asked my current EP about the wisdom of a big dose at this point, I *know* she would have vetoed the idea. There had been signs already that my once efficient anti-arrhythmic medication was now doing too good a job at slowing down my electrical heart signals.

I can't remember checking inside that day—closing my eyes, quieting my mind, and asking for guidance from deep within. Somehow, in my eagerness to cut through the seemingly endless frustration of recovery, I had skipped over that promise to myself. Now I've come to believe more than ever that we need to trust our gut assessment on any important matter. By not checking within, I was not honoring my body the morning I took the dangerous dose. Nor did I check with a health professional. What a way to learn a lesson!

Emotional Ups and Downs
As my own experience attests, mood swings are a huge part of the recovery picture, and they can be very disconcerting. Every cell in a heart surgery patient's body has received a call to arms. Head and heart will need time to realign because a powerful body shake-up has occurred. Thus I've come to believe that the depression reaction following surgery is partly physiological.

At the very least, our emotions are fragile. While not a news junkie, I have been a National Public Radio regular. But suddenly I couldn't bear to hear its in-depth postwar reporting on Iraq, or about yet another suicide bomb attack in Jerusalem. I was simply feeling too vulnerable, and so music became my preferred listening alternative. Several weeks passed before I listened to news reporting of any kind again, and I was highly selective regarding print news as well.

Nor was I capable of entertaining conversation whose energy was not positive. I remember one run-in on the phone with a family member who wanted to tease me about the gory details of surgery soon after I was home. Perhaps he meant well. But I was feeling far too close to it all and had to terminate the conversation on the spot.

Sometimes, it seems, these emotional ups and downs have even more dramatic consequences. In the course of my research I encountered two patients who manifested a temporary change of character. One sixty-eight-year-old man I spoke with was apparently inconsolable as he navigated his post-bypass challenges. He became angry and mean-spirited, repeatedly complaining that there was nothing his wife could do right to ease his constant distress, and according to her, being nasty was completely out of character for him. Another patient, a woman in her fifties, confided to me six weeks after her valve replacement that she "hadn't been nice to anyone" since. Simply put, even a strongly held resolve to maintain a positive, proactive attitude can melt away. (*A note for caregivers:* While ignoring the occasional irritable outburst comes with the territory, tolerating nastiness does not. Caregivers have every right to expect appreciation and cooperation from the people they are caring for, and should stand up for themselves in the face of abusive behavior. See "Caring for Yourself" on pages 63–64.)

Here's a composite snapshot on the blues: For the first four to six weeks after your operation, you can expect tears to flow for no specific reason. You can expect to wake up in the morning feeling down, even temporarily hopeless, and to experience setbacks and reversals in addition to positive progress forward. But remember, the operative word here is *temporarily.* Things will change. You *will* go back to feeling your true self again.

In the meantime, what can you do to dispel a dismal mood? In my case, I've found that regularly reviewing what I have to be grateful for in life can dissolve tension and negativity. I feel much better after reminding myself of all my blessings—my soul mate Bill, my children, Bill's children, their partners in life, our grandchildren, our entire family's level of good health, the blessed environment in which I live. By simply saying thank you, even out loud, as I consciously visualize the abundance in my life, I am restored and renewed.

If depressive episodes are running you more than you are on top of them, *discuss your symptoms with your health-care professional.* If they are instead transient and intermittent, here are some diversions and coping strategies to try:

- Take a walk in the fresh air. Combat lethargy. Force yourself to get exercise despite your fatigue.
- Find a good book, or a trashy one, that fully engages you; don't try too hard to cover "important" material.
- Explore meditation. Try sitting in peaceful solitude and following your breath, for even five minutes a day.
- Go into prayer. (The Fall 2004 issue of *Journal of Health Psychology* reports on ongoing research by Amy Ai and her colleagues, "pioneers in the new field of

positive psychology" at the University of Michigan, to identify a mechanism that triggers the "faith effect" in patients undergoing open-heart surgery.)

- Search out things that tickle your funny bone. A compendium of jokes? *Comedy Central? Saturday Night Live?*
- Listen to your favorite upbeat music.
- Bake a cake or cook a meal with a friend (rest when you get tired).
- Exchange supportive phone calls with another heart patient. Swapping experiences is especially valuable in putting smaller questions to rest.
- Sit in the sunshine; take in a view.
- Don't play Lone Ranger. Ask for help! Call on old friends, as well as new ones.
- Review your prescription mix with your doctor.
- Discuss taking a sleeping remedy or an antidepressant for the short term.

Beginning a Cardiac Rehab Program—Eureka!

Some patients are healed enough to begin a cardiac rehabilitation program—which I highly recommend—sooner, some later. Two months after my surgery, I was cleared to begin a physician-sponsored program based in a gym facility where I live in Santa Fe, called the Center for Living Well, which is spaciously housed in the basement of our one hospital. Since over the last thirty years thousands of such programs have sprung up nationwide, there's probably one near you as well.

Here are some highlights of my experience. I was finally up to moving my body for real. I knew I had made tangible progress or I wouldn't have been referred to the Center by my doctor. I was assigned an exercise physiologist, or case manager. After a general orientation (involving completing a detailed questionnaire, learning to take my own pulse, and understanding rhythm monitoring guidelines), I was given a personal exercise worksheet. Preferably three times a week for one hour, I was to track my gentle progress forward in a customized program—using the treadmill, bike, stairs, UBE machine (aerobic ergometer), and so on. Adding weight training to the regimen was to come later, at the discretion of my case manager. In addition, numerous classes (stretching, therabands, free weights) and support groups (smoking cessation, stress management, osteoporosis and diet education) were all available in the package. Once a month an "Ask the Cardiologist" question-and-answer session was also offered, hosted by one of the New Mexico Heart Institute's cardiologists. Best of all, the staff was made up of caring, devoted, highly attentive, and good-humored professionals. There also was a palpable sense of camaraderie in the air, inspiring patients who saw one another regularly to develop friendships and become members of a de facto support group.

I was accepted into the program provided I agreed to wear a wireless heart monitor during exercise. What a good thing! My heart was still ricocheting in and out of an irregular rhythm, but there was always someone at a computer screen monitoring for rhythm changes. If, as is more likely with exertion, my atrial fib returned, even if I didn't notice, a nurse or exercise physiologist would check in with me. How was I feeling? Was I lightheaded? Did I need to slow down? Maybe end my session for the day? "Your pulse is such-and-such. Let's check your blood pressure..." (Since a patient's inclination may be to push through—my common approach in the past—the permission to simply stop, give yourself a break, can be welcome.) I felt completely taken care of. With so many dedicated professionals around me, and the new friends I was making, I could never run into too much trouble. Although physically challenging at times, the cardiac rehab environment made for a positive, confidence-restoring experience.

In the book *Heart Attack! Advice for Patients by Patients,* most of the eleven contributors go out of their way to rave about their cardiac rehab program experience: "The highlight of my day," "I credit the program with getting my life back on track," "I've been a member now for ten years and I know it is keeping me healthy," "My wife is now in the program with me. We've made some great friends." The social and emotional support received can be so valuable that even after they are ready to return to previous gym or yoga classes, many heart patients continue to take advantage of their ongoing membership in a cardio-directed program.

Planning for the Future

Staying well for the long-term is now your goal. Toward that end, what will matter most is making conscious choices for an appropriate lifestyle. A general recommendation is to avoid compartmentalizing this or that risk factor as your exclusive focus—lowering cholesterol, say, or quitting smoking, cutting down on saturated fat, increasing exercise. Think instead in terms of total lifestyle choices that will give you energy, joy, and well-being in the future.

This includes finding an accessible physician you can be comfortable with and trust over the next decades. At this point you are looking for long-term continuity of care, someone who will listen to you, hear your fears, and treat you with respect. Here are some guidelines to help you choose the right physician for you:

- Investigate doctors in your community. Choose a primary care physician, and plan on occasional visits to a cardiologist. Or your first choice may be a cardiologist, or an osteopath, or another medical professional.
- Get personal feedback or referrals from friends and members of any support group you have contacted.
- Ask the surgeon who performed your procedure to recommend a practitioner for your long-term care.
- Have these conversations as soon as you can, even as you are regaining your health and strength. Don't wait for an emergency situation before seeking out a medical team you can trust.

Practicing Persistent Self-Care
Here are words of recuperative wisdom from Dr. Linda McNamar, which appeared in the January 2004 issue of *Science of Mind* magazine:

There's an old proverb which says, "You cannot prevent the birds of unhappiness from flying over your head, but you can prevent them from making a nest in your hair." When we are ill, we may feel lost as to what to do or where to go. Waiting may have the feel of being passive, but think of the caterpillar in the cocoon, the seed in the ground, or a mother bird sitting on her egg. Waiting in our lostness is sometimes vital for the journey into wholeness.

The most important caring you can do for yourself, before and after surgery, is to make the choice to put yourself first. Choose to care for your every need and desire—for your body, for your mind, for your spirit. Make your needs known, from having a truth-telling discussion with a loved one to placing that extra phone call to your health professional.

Above all, give yourself a daily gift of hope. Compose a new affirmation of gratitude *for yourself*—one to revisit and perhaps revise every day—for the gift of your life. Here's how mine began:

I am healing well, one day at a time.
All is beautiful and all is well in my world.
I see the results of my healing every day.
Soon I will be back hiking the beautiful Santa Fe trails.
I celebrate my life and my heart's restored health!

Use your recovery as a time to get to know yourself better, and to deepen your connection with the human and natural worlds that surround you. Think lovingly about yourself and your life-changing experience—write about it, share it with others.

EPILOGUE

Three Journal Entries

*The great thing about life is that as long as we live
we have the privilege of growing.*

—Joshua Loth Liebman

THESE ARE ENTRIES I RECORDED in my journal as I passed key
milestones on the journey to "return to my old self"—or should
I say, discovering a new one.

Six Months After Surgery

January 16, 2004

Through my open-heart surgery experience I have
been given a wonderful gift: pristine new life energy.
I am so happy with where my life is right now. As if
I am infused with deep multicolored ribbons of
meaning—blue, green, pink, red—I feel purposeful

on many levels. The writer in me has joyfully resurfaced after several years. I've felt called to write on the open-heart surgery encounter to share a life-changing experience and to support others.

Until my need for surgery, it never crossed my mind that such a role was ahead of me. Yet it's clear now that, from the day I was born, this unique assignment to benefit others was set in motion.

Like Dr. Eric Pearl, whose teleconference I participated in this morning, my life has new meaning. I zealously appreciate the time I have here on the planet, the joyful and healthy full life I lead right now...

I know that my life is going exactly as it's meant to be going, that I am getting on with the work I am meant to be doing.

The month of January 2004 has progressed with ease. I've been so content to be in this beautiful spirit-laden environment, even though January is our coldest month. Numerous publishing coaching clients are appearing, and I am up to it! I've benefited enormously from my cardiac rehab program. I have started up my Korean yoga classes again. I'm pleased to return to the balanced practice of invigorating movement and peace, all in one hour of class twice a week.

What have I learned? To follow the energy... I am stronger than I have been in two or three years. My vitality is back. Everything is working. I am so blessed.

Eight Months After Surgery
March 9, 2004

My view of myself is shifting back to "normal." By that I mean I am seeing myself as a non–medically challenged person once again. I have been thrilled with the terrific cardiac rehab gym program I've attended. I "graduated" from Phase II, a course of 36 sessions, a month ago. I no longer have to suit up with a wireless heart monitor to be followed for atrial fibrillation during exercise. If I like, I can continue to use this gym at the hospital indefinitely.

I've grown particularly fond of the weight machines—equipment like the chest press, the seated leg press, the lat pull, the overhead press—none of which I'd used before. I had carried around the notion that the weight machine scene was simply not for me. I could feel my body atrophy day by day in the early weeks of recovery even though I labored to increase my walking. With hindsight, I see it was the ongoing low-grade fever and anemia that was holding me back. So when I was finally fit enough to begin the gym program at about nine weeks, I was ecstatic.

However, now, many weeks later, between my biweekly anticoagulant-monitoring appointments and two or three workout sessions per week at the gym, I've been seeing much too much of St. Vincent Hospital. I've parked my car *for five months* now in the hospital's parking lot. I'm tired of seeing myself as medically challenged. Except for inconsequential brief episodes of atrial fibrillation, I am back to being a vibrant, perky spirit! So I want a change from this medical center's gym.

I am a youthful sixty-two now. I am trim, attractive, sexy. I am too vain to stop coloring my hair…one of my most attractive assets. Yes, my face is showing signs of age. I don't like that. But in sum, I love my youthful bounce and appearance and do not intend to let that go.

Heart or lung patients at the hospital's gym move a lot slower than I do….As a whole, the rehab crowd is a decelerated, much older population that continues to attend the Center for Living Well at St. Vincent. It's a genuinely supportive program and I'm happy to be able to recommend it. It's just that now, eight months past my own open-heart surgery, I identify much more with the gang at my old yoga center, where yoga practitioners are equally represented from their thirties through their seventies. I also plan to investigate a new gym to continue the weight training.

One Year Anniversary After Surgery!

July 16, 2004

It is only now, in the last few months, as I have let go of worry and become fully healed, that I realize how underprepared I was to meet the psychological stress of heart surgery. My continuing frustration with atrial fib, after expecting it to dissipate three months following the open-heart operation, delayed my recovery. I did not fit neatly into the 80–20% statistic. I didn't land in the 80% group whose a-fib magically vanishes after three months. Plus, I'm a survivor in her sixties of this rare congenital heart defect, and no studies or statistics *exist* in the medical archives for a much older "Ebsteiner." I continue to chart my own course.

A great learning for me has been to realize the merit in stepping back, of taking more contemplative time to evaluate any situation, including my health. After choosing the surgical route, I became fixated on getting through the operation, and affirming positive postsurgery outcomes. Nothing wrong with that. Except that I didn't let it dawn on me deeply enough that there was an afterward. Given my underlying state of anxiety, I'm not sure I could have welcomed an additional step-by-step roadmap through the recovery process in advance. The surgical process was plenty to focus on! Yet had someone taken me aside and emphasized how *advance* knowledge is power I would have suffered less…[from] weakness and fatigue, debilitating anemia, aggravating constipation, and the onset of pericarditis in the guise of an ordinary virus…. I've now learned that educating ourselves before-hand minimizes anxiety, frustration, even depression, and paves the way for a speedier, more self-confident recovery.

I believe my put-on-a-happy-face front hindered more frank communication with my surgeon and his team. I was so eager to appear "fine" in the hospital that I created my own doctor-patient communication gap….

Today my atrial fib has finally become minimal. Some days I think to myself: it's nonexistent. It's too soon, undoubtedly, to make that claim and to go off the anticoagulant, Coumadin. However, one year later I can truly say I have moved on from my tricuspid valve "makeover" experience. I have a faint scar. That's what shows. My gusto for living has fully returned. That really shows! I affirm my gratitude for my health and my life every morning—every day.

Guidelines and Checklists

Use the entries that follow as guidelines for constructing your own lists of things to do and issues to resolve, both before your surgery and during your period of recovery.

Think of the checklists as assignments. Include space for notes (with dates) as you address each issue, and give yourself tentative deadlines where appropriate.

More detail is available in the chapters cross-referenced here. Also, an extensive, nine-page Recovery Organizer is available for downloading on my website: www.openheartcoach.com.

Remember: Advance knowledge is power.

First Steps (see Chapters 1 and 2)

❏ Designate an advocate-caregiver who will accompany you before, during, and after surgery (see Chapter 2 on care for the caregiver).

❏ Select the surgeon; get a second opinion.

❏ Choose a hospital.

❏ Check surgeon and hospital quality at www.healthgrades.com.

❏ Arrange a meeting with your anesthesiologist, if possible, at least twenty-four hours before surgery.

❏ Cultivate a positive attitude (see "An Exercise for Overcoming Fear and Envisioning Hope" on pages 48–49).

❏ Get your affairs in order as time permits:
    Update your living trust or will.
    Review instructions regarding beneficiaries, powers of attorney, and a living will.
    Prepare a list citing the locations of important documents.

Preparing for Surgery (see Chapters 3, 4, and 5)

❏ Draw up questions for the medical team and get answers to them.

❏ Compile your own medical fact sheet with details of your upcoming surgery.

❏ Make a calendar for scheduling forthcoming tests and appointments needed before surgery.

❏ Locate and begin a daily prepare-for-surgery program.

❏ Begin a daily journal.

❏ Join a local or online support group.

❏ Give consideration to what your level of functioning will be once you go home (see Chapter 5).

❏ Decide whether to seek short-term counseling.

As the Date Approaches (see Chapters 3, 6, and 7)

❑ Request take-home instructions and review them with a physician's assistant.

❑ Watch the hospital's educational video to get a solid sense of what will go on (see also Chapter 7).

❑ Download information on postsurgery day-by-day hospital care from the Cleveland Clinic's website (www.cleveland-clinic.org) or your own hospital's website.

❑ Prepare for your hospital stay and pack your suitcase (see Chapter 6):

Collect CDs of calming music; as well as a good new book or magazines; inquire about coping strategies for heart surgery recovery from family members or friends.

Compose a list of affirmations and read them daily.

Choose the music or healing affirmations you will use under anesthesia on the day of your surgery.

Consider arranging for Therapeutic Touch (TT) at the hospital.

Anticipating and Managing Recovery (see Chapters 4, 5, 8, 9, and 10)

❏ Educate yourself about the ups and downs of recovery: Consult your healthcare team about what to expect.

Ask for advice from friends who've been through major surgery or members of your support group.

Check the "Resources" section of this book for other sources of information.

Expect the pace of your recovery to be uneven.

❏ Organize a "home team" to help you with: Meals and shopping

Household chores

Driving

Updating friends and family about your progress via a group email list or phone-call chain

❏ Ask your medical team for a list of issues to watch for once you're home (do this *before* you leave the hospital), including those that would prompt a call to 911.

❏ Make a list of phone numbers to call for questions or concerns, including contacts to phone at night or on weekends.

❏ Get detailed information (*before* you leave the hospital) about the medications you'll be taking during your recovery.

❏ Set up a journal in which you can record your progress. (This will be useful if you need help with snags or set-backs in your recovery.)

❏ Prepare a calendar to keep track of follow-up appointments.

❏ Line up sources of psychological and spiritual support.

❏ Find the best doctor to advise you during the years ahead.

Glossary

Ablation. Elimination or removal of abnormal rhythm, usually by "ablating," or burning out, the abnormal area in the heart.

Adult congenital cardiologist. A medical doctor who specializes in the diagnosis and treatment of adults with heart disorders that have been present since birth.

Angiogram. An X-ray picture (angiography) of the blood flow in an artery or vein, used to examine the heart's circulatory system. See *Catheterization.*

Anticoagulant. Medicine that delays clotting of the blood by suppressing production of the enzyme thrombin.

Arrhythmia. An abnormal heart rhythm.

Atrial fibrillation. One type of irregular heart rhythm originating in the heart's upper chambers (the atria). The formation of blood clots is a common problem associated with **atrial fib**, or **a-fib**, which is why anticoagulants are frequently prescribed. See *Anticoagulant.*

Atrial flutter. A less-concerning but nevertheless irritable irregular heart rhythm.

Blood transfusion. The providing of blood to a person in need of additional blood—for example, during or following surgery.

Breastbone. The vertical bone in the front and center of the chest, to which the ribs are connected; also called the sternum.

Cardiac rehab program. A program of exercise and risk-factor education for individuals recovering from serious heart procedures and heart disease.

Cardiovascular diseases (CVD). Diseases related to, or involving, the heart and blood vessels.

Cardioversion. The process of converting an abnormal heart rhythm to a normal one.

Catheterization. A diagnostic procedure during which small tubes called catheters are inserted into the body to measure pressure and blood flow in the heart.

Echocardiogram. A noninvasive test in which pulses of sound are sent into the body and the echoes returning from the beating heart produce images that are recorded. The procedure is used to measure the size of the heart's four chambers, to examine the heart valves, to assess heart function, and more.

Electrophysiologist (EP). A cardiologist who specializes in the heart's electrical functions.

Emergency room (ER). The unit of a healthcare facility that provides rapid emergency treatment for people with sudden illness or trauma.

Endocarditis. Inflammation of the thin inner membrane that lines the heart muscle or its valves.

Heart block. A type of arrhythmia that results in serious slowing or blocking of the electrical impulses seeking to reach the pumping chambers of the heart.

Heart-lung machine. A machine through which blood is temporarily diverted, to keep oxygenated blood moving through the body during open-heart surgery. The machine maintains circulation until the heart and lungs are able to return to normal functioning.

Heart monitor. A device for monitoring and recording heart rhythms.

Intensive care unit (ICU). A hospital unit with high-tech equipment, monitoring devices, and medical and nursing staff who provide specialized care, especially following surgery.

Irregular heart rhythm. Heartbeat that is unpredictable and without pattern; also called arrhythmia.

Mitral valve. One of the heart's valves, composed of two triangular flaps, located between the upper and lower chambers on the left side of the heart.

Operating room (OR). The highly specialized unit in the hospital equipped for performing surgical operations.

Pericarditis. Inflammation of the sac that encloses the heart.

Regurgitation. The flowing backwards of blood—for example, when the blood travels back through a particular heart valve rather than continuing forward along its normal route.

Right atrium. One of the two upper heart chambers, this one on the right side of the chest.

Sinus rhythm. The medical name for normal heart rhythm.

Sternum. The vertical bone in the front and center of the chest to which ribs are connected; also called the breastbone.

Telemetry. The technology for monitoring, sending, and receiving data from one location to another.

Therapeutic Touch (TT). A calming, healing procedure, done without actually touching the body, that can be provided by a specially trained TT nurse.

Tricuspid valve. The valve between the upper and lower chambers on the right side of the heart, consisting of three flaps of tissue, that keeps the blood from flowing back up and into the right atrium.

Valve displacement. An abnormal structural placement of a heart valve.

Ventilator. A respirator or breathing device.

Resources

Recent Books

Burrows, S., and C. Gassert, *Moving Right Along after Open-Heart Surgery* (Atlanta: Pritchett & Hull Associates, 1996).

Cardiac Therapy Foundation of the Midpeninsula, *Heart Attack! Advice for Patients by Patients*, edited by K. Berra, et al (New Haven: Yale University Press, 2002).

Cohan, C., J. B. Pimm, and J. R. Jude, *Coping with Heart Surgery and Bypassing Depression: A Family's Guide to the Medical, Emotional, and Practical Issues,* 3rd ed. (Madison, Connecticut: Psychosocial Press, 1998).

Farquhar, J. W., and G. A. Spiller, *Diagnosis: Heart Disease—Answers to Your Questions about Recovery and Lasting Health* (New York: W.W. Norton, 2001).

Gould, K. L., *Heal Your Heart: How You Can Prevent or Reverse Heart Disease* (New Brunswick, New Jersey: Rutgers University Press, 1998).

Hillman, J., *The Thought of the Heart and the Soul of the World* (Dallas, Texas: Spring Publications, 1992).

Kligfield, P., and M. Seaton, *The Cardiac Recovery Handbook: The Complete Guide to Life after Heart Attack or Heart Surgery* (New York: Hatherleigh Press, 2004).

Mailhot, C., M. Brubaker, and L. Slezak, *Surgery: A Patient's Guide from Diagnosis to Recovery* (San Francisco: UCSF Nursing Press, 1999).

McTaggart, L., *The Field: The Quest for the Secret Force of the Universe* (New York: HarperCollins, 2003).

Mayo Clinic Heart Book: The Ultimate Guide to Heart Health, rev. ed. (New York: William Morrow, 2000).

Neugeboren, J., *Open Heart: A Patient's Story of Life-Saving Medicine and Life-Giving Friendship* (New York: Houghton Mifflin, 2003).

Oz, M., *Healing from the Heart: A Leading Surgeon Combines Eastern and Western Traditions to Create the Medicine of the Future* (New York: Plume, 1999).

Pearsall, P., *The Heart's Code: Tapping the Wisdom and Power of Our Heart Energy—The New Findings about Cellular Memories and Their Role in the Mind / Body / Spirit Connection* (New York: Broadway Books, 1998).

Sotile, W. M., with R. Cantor-Cooke, *Thriving with Heart Disease: A Unique Program for You and Your Family—Live Happier, Healthier, Longer* (New York: Free Press, 2003).

Older Books of Note

Richards, N., *Heart to Heart: A Cleveland Clinic Guide to Understanding Heart Disease and Open-Heart Surgery* (New York: Atheneum, 1987).

Waxberg, J., *Bypass: A Doctor's Recovery from Open-Heart Surgery* (New York: Appleton-Century-Crofts, 1981).

Coping Techniques

Albert, I., and Z. Keithley, *Write Yourself Well: Journal Your Self to Health* (Whitefish, Montana: Mountain Greenery Press, 2004).

Benson, H., and M. Klipper, *The Relaxation Response* (New York: Avon Books, 1976). "A simple meditative technique that has helped millions to cope with fatigue, anxiety, and stress."

Huddleston, P., *Prepare for Surgery, Heal Faster: A Guide of Mind-Body Techniques* (Cambridge, Massachusetts: Angel River Press, 1996). CD or audiotape sold separately.

Naperstek, B., *A Meditation to Promote a Successful Surgery* (Akron, Ohio: Health Journeys, 1992). A two-tape set.

Pearl, E., *The Reconnection: Heal Others, Heal Yourself* (Carlsbad, California: Hay House, 2004).

Professional and Government Organizations

Adult Congenital Heart Association
www.achaheart.org

American Heart Association
www.americanheart.org

Cleveland Clinic
www.clevelandclinic.org

Mayo Clinic
www.mayoclinic.org

Mended Hearts
www.mendedhearts.org

National Heart, Lung, and Blood Institute
www.nhlbi.nih.gov

Health Newsletters

Harvard Heart Letter
www.health.harvard.edu

Mayo Clinic Women's Healthsource
www.mayoclinic.org

Nutrition Action Health Letter
www.cspinet.org

More Online Resources

www.aftermybypass.org

www.ChoiceTrust.com

www.Healthfinder.gov

www.HealthGrades.com

www.HeartCenterOnline.com

www.HeartInfo.org

www.HospitalCompare.hhs.gov

www.LeapFrogGroup.org/cp

www.MedHelp.com

www.MedlinePlus.gov

www.openheartcoach.com

www.WebMD.com

Acknowledgments

This book would not have been possible were it not for fellow travelers with "miles and miles and miles of heart"—patients and caregivers, medical providers, advance readers, dear friends, professional coaching buddies, and most of all, my loving family. I give thanks to all of you who have been there for me during and beyond my adventure with open-heart surgery. You have helped make *The Open Heart Companion* a reality.

Thank you, first, to the magnificent staff at the Mayo Clinic in Rochester, Minnesota. My Mayo Clinic team—my superb cardiothoracic surgeon, Joseph Dearani, MD; adult congenital heart specialist Nasar Ammash, MD; Stephen Hammill, MD, director of heart rhythm services; and physician's assistant Lucinda Stroetz. Lucinda was one of three cardiac surgery specialists who provided my manuscript with invaluable suggestions. Special heartfelt thanks to the team of caring nurses in the OR, the ICU, and on the coronary care unit at Saint Marys Hospital, also in Rochester.

Closer to home it is Kathy Blake, MD, a cardiologist at the New Mexico Heart Institute in Albuquerque, to whom I will be forever grateful. She insisted I consult the congenital heart specialists at the Mayo Clinic, world-renowned for treating my rare structural heart problem. Thank you also to Grant La Farge, MD, a pediatric cardiologist in Santa Fe, whose specialty has been Ebstein's Anomaly. Although the reality check that he once delivered to me—that one day I might have to have my valve "fixed"—landed on deaf ears at first, he sounded the warning that open-heart surgery down the road was a distinct possibility.

Although it's now two and a half years later, I want to acknowledge my wonderful home team—a group of eleven close friends and neighbors who were corralled into service by my terrific organizer friend, Paula Heffner. All these dear ones either brought dinner, chauffeured, ran errands, or checked in by phone for weeks during my recovery: Satsuki Annino, Mary Lou Capper, Charlotte Cockman, Ilona Klein, Nancy Kreger, Katie Lopez, Michelle Morgan, Rebecca Skeele, Sharon Spence, and Hannah Wilder. Most of all, I am very grateful to my daughter-in-law, Meredith Fein Lichtenberg, for the remarkable suggestion to organize a home team in the first place.

I am indebted to several readers and commentators who provided feedback at the very beginning of this project, especially Denys Cope, RN; Angela Campos; Jim Preus; Sherry James; and Ruby Auburg. Special thanks to my son Greg Lichtenberg, my daughter Amanda Lichtenberg, and my daughter-in-law Yance Ford, who provided me with constant encouragement.

I also offer deep appreciation and praise to the more than sixty heart patients and caregivers who agreed to be interviewed for this book: I have learned so much from you. I am grateful as well for extended commentary shared during the free monthly phone support groups established through my website; in particular, enormous thanks for final manuscript readings by several heart patients and caregivers, including Beth Philips Brown, Jo Anne Esfahani, Richard Rossbauer, Jodi Spafford, and Lloyd Vansant. And finally thanks to Angela de Albuquerque, RN, BSN, at the Heart Center at Doylestown Hospital near Philadelphia, for finding me on the Internet, for her helpful manuscript reading, and for offering to locate former heart patient volunteers at the Heart Center to review and comment, as well.

To my life coaching buddies with whom I meet over the phone twice a month—Marsha Lehman, Siobhan Murphy, and Michele Christensen—thank you for your loving support and long partnership. Thanks also to a wonderful business coach, Karyn Greenstreet, whose wise counsel helped me establish a highly successful Internet presence in launching my website, www.openheartcoach.com. And a very warm thanks to Cheryl Richardson, who has been an enthusiastic supporter of my open heart coaching service.

It is with deep gratitude and appreciation that I thank those who have been partners on my book publication team. First, with extra special gratitude, I give thanks to Marilyn Abraham, whose early editorial guidance was so grounding in shaping this book. Thanks to Chris Kochansky, who is one of the most talented editors I know. Thanks to Ellen Kleiner of Blessingway Authors' Services, who shepherded *The Open Heart Companion* through the production process with thoughtful suggestions and support. Thanks to designer Janice St. Marie, who contributed her heartfelt creative touch.

Thanks, finally, to my husband Bill, whose unconditional love and support is a blessed and cherished gift.

And most important, I am immeasurably grateful to the loving Higher Power for my life, to mother-father God who guides my life and provided me with the mission to deliver this book.

Index

About the Author

Maggie Lichtenberg's nine-year-old coaching business is unique because she serves two very different communities. First, as a former editorial, marketing, and sales publishing company executive for twenty years in New York and Boston, she maintains a private practice as a publishing coach and consultant. Her new direction has evolved out of her experience with unexpected open-heart surgery in July 2003.

Now thriving, Maggie has a passion to support open-heart patients (709,000 people undergo open-heart surgery in this country each year) and their caregivers to plan ahead for the challenging two-to-three-month recovery period at home. A professional speaker and international facilitator for the past fifteen years, Maggie now is an open heart coach to heart patients and their loved ones, presenting her educational support programs at medical facilities and heart-related conferences, as well as leading monthly phone support groups on practical home recovery.

An author as well, Maggie's essays, criticism, and magazine features have appeared in such national publications as *The New York Times Book Review, Publishers Weekly, The Nation, Ms., Mademoiselle, Hope,* and *Working Woman.* She has been listed in *Who's Who in America* and in *Who's Who of American Women* for many years. She received her BA from the University of Michigan, and pursued graduate work at Harvard University on a Woodrow Wilson Fellowship. She also is past president of the New York Chapter of the Women's National Book Association.

Maggie has two adult children, both published writers, living in New York City. She currently resides in Santa Fe, New Mexico, with her husband Bill.

Learn more about Maggie's publishing coaching at www.maggielichtenberg.com and about her open heart patient and caregiver support programs at www.openheartcoach.com. To subscribe to her free online newsletter, *Heart To Heart,* send a blank email message to HeartToHeart-On@zines.webvalence.com.

ORDER FORM

Quantity   **Amount**

_____ *The Open Heart Companion: Preparation*
and Guidance for Open-Heart Surgery
Recovery ($20.00)   _____

Sales tax of 6.3125% for NM residents   _____

Shipping & handling
($5.00 for first book; $1.50
for each additional book)   _____

Total amount enclosed   _____
Bulk purchase discounts available.

Method of payment

❏ Check or money order enclosed (payable to Open Heart
  Publishing, in US funds only)
❏ MasterCard   ❏ VISA

CREDIT CARD #: _____ EXP _____

SIGNATURE: _____

Ship to (please print):

NAME _____

ADDRESS _____

CITY/STATE/ZIP _____

PHONE _____

OPEN HEART
PUBLISHING

4 Cosmos Court, Santa Fe, NM 87508-2285
phone toll free: 866-986-8807 fax: 505-986-8794
www.openheartcoach.com